Women's Health During and After Pregnancy

A Theory-Based Study of Adaptation to Change

Lorraine Tulman, DNSc, RN, FAAN, is an Associate Professor at the University of Pennsylvania School of Nursing.

Jacqueline Fawcett, PhD, RN, FAAN, is a Professor in the College of Nursing and Health Sciences at the University of Massachusetts–Boston.

Women's Health During and After Pregnancy

A Theory-Based Study of Adaptation to Change

Lorraine Tulman, DNSc, RN, FAAN
Jacqueline Fawcett, PhD, RN, FAAN

 Springer Publishing Company

Copyright © 2003 by Springer Publishing Company, Inc.

Springer Publishing Company, Inc.
536 Broadway
New York, NY 10012-3955

Acquisitions Editor: Ruth Chasek
Production Editor: J. Hurkin-Torres
Cover design by Joanne Honigman

03 04 05 06 07 / 5 4 3 2 1

Library of Congress Cataloging-in-Publication Data

Tulman, Lorraine.
  Women's health during and after pregnancy : a theory-based study of adaptation to change / Lorraine Tulman, Jacqueline Fawcett.
      p. ; cm.
  Includes bibliographical references and index.
  ISBN 0-8261-1994-8
  1. Pregnancy. 2. Childbirth. 3. Obstetrics. 4. Women—Health and hygiene. I. Fawcett, Jacqueline. II. Title.
  [DNLM: 1. Pregnancy. 2. Adaptation, Psychological.
3. Delivery. 4. Puerperium. 5. Women's Health.
WQ 200 T923w 2003]
RG525 .T85 2003
618.2—dc21   2002070497
                                                    CIP

Printed in the United States of America by Sheridan Books.

To Alan, for your encouragement, wisdom, and love.

—LT

To John, for your love, understanding of the demands of my work, and the creation of an environment in which I can enjoy the challenges of conducting research and preparing the results for publication.

—JF

Contents

Preface

Childbearing typically is characterized as a period of good health for most women in the United States. Despite this fact, medical and nursing textbooks describe the time after delivery as one of recovery from childbearing, thereby implying that pregnancy and delivery are illnesses. We believe that a more accurate perspective is that of adaptation. In particular, we view both pregnancy and the postpartum as times of considerable and often profound change requiring adaptation.

In this book, we describe the results of a National Institute for Nursing Research, National Institutes of Health-funded longitudinal study of women's health during pregnancy and the postpartum—including physical and psychosocial health, functional status, and family relationships—based in the Roy Adaptation Model (Grant Number RO1-NR02340). More specifically, we present a detailed description of how women's physical health, psychosocial health, and family relationships are related to their usual household, social and community, child care, occupational, educational, and personal care activities, that is, their functional status during pregnancy and the postpartum. The study participants included more than 200 women whom we followed throughout the three trimesters of pregnancy and the first six postpartum months.

The study was an outcome of our longstanding commitment to enhancing understanding of women's health during life transitions, with childbearing as the prototype for women's adaptation during a normal life transition. Our journey to this study began when we recognized the need for an instrument to measure functioning as an outcome for a study of the effects of antepartum information on women's adaptation to unplanned Cesarean birth. The subsequent construction and psychometric testing of the Inventory of Functional Status After Childbirth was the beginning of a research program designed to examine women's functioning during the childbearing period. The study described in this book presents the largest of the studies in our research program to date and represents an extension of our thinking from a relatively narrow focus on functioning to a broader focus on women's health and adaptation during the normal life transition of childbearing, including both pregnancy and the postpartum.

We believe that nurse researchers have an obligation to identify the implications of their study findings for nursing practice and the formulation of health policies. Accordingly, we explain how the data obtained from the healthy women who participated in our study may be used to develop nursing interventions that may facilitate optimal functional status during pregnancy and the postpartum. We also explain how the results of this study have supplied data that can help shape legislation concerning state and national maternity leave/compensation policies. Indeed, the critical information provided by the women in our study could place discussions about the length of maternity leave on an empirical rather than an intuitive basis.

We have divided the book into five parts. We introduce the reader to our study in Part I. In chapter 1, we explain our Theory of Adaptation During Childbearing, describe its derivation from the Roy Adaptation Model, and identify the specific study variables.

We focus on women's adaptation during pregnancy in Part II. In chapter 2, we describe the results of our study dealing with women's performance of usual household, social and community, child care, personal care, occupational, and educational activities, as well as their reports of levels of physical energy and physical symptoms experienced during the three trimesters of pregnancy. In chapter 3, we report the results of our study dealing with the relation of prepregnancy weight and weight gain during pregnancy to functional status, physical symptoms, and physical energy during each trimester of pregnancy. In chapter 4, we present our study results dealing with psychosocial health, family relationships, and functional status during the three trimesters of pregnancy.

We focus on adaptation after delivery in Part III. In chapter 5, we report the results of our study dealing with women's performance of usual household, social and community, infant care, child care, personal care, occupational, and educational activities, as well as their reports of levels of physical energy and physical symptoms experienced during the first six months after delivery. In chapter 6, we present our data on women's weight during the first six postpartum months, along with the relation of postpartum weight to physical symptoms and physical energy. We also consider the influence of infant feeding method on postpartum weight. In chapter 7, we describe our study results for psychosocial health, family relationships, maternal perception of infant temperament, infant nocturnal sleep, and functional status during the first six months of the postpartum. We also describe restrictions on the women's activity after delivery, the women's support systems, and the help with child care they had when they returned to work or school.

Each chapter of Part II and Part III includes a summary of the relevant theoretical and empirical literature, as well as the results of our analyses of the quantitative data we obtained from questionnaires and the qualitative data we obtained from an in-depth interview of each woman conducted at six months after delivery. In each of these chapters, our analyses include descriptions of changes, as well as correlational data for relations of physical health variables or psychosocial health variables and family relationships variables with functional status during each trimester of pregnancy or at three and six weeks and three and six months postpartum. We augment the quantitative data in each chapter with qualitative data from our interviews with the women at six months postpartum. In addition, we place the literature and the data within the context of the Roy Adaptation Model and our Theory of Adaptation During Childbearing.

We finish the presentation of our study results in Part IV. In chapter 8, we present our analysis of the women's recollections of their childbearing experiences from the vantage point of six months after delivery, along with their recommendations for lifestyle adjustments that can facilitate adaptation during pregnancy and the postpartum. In chapter 9, we discuss how the data provided by the women who participated in our study can be used to develop clinical interventions that may facilitate optimal functional status and adaptation throughout the childbearing period, as well as the implications of our study results for further development of maternity leave policy.

We conclude the book in Part V. In chapter 10, we revisit our Theory of Adaptation During Childbearing. Here, we summarize the study results and discuss the empirical adequacy of the theory. We also discuss the utility and credibility of the Roy Adaptation Model for research with childbearing women.

The reader who wishes more detail about the study methodology may refer to the Appendix, which includes a detailed description of the study sample and methodology. The Appendix also includes a table listing the definition of each study variable and the instrument used to measure each variable.

This book was written for baccalaureate, master's and doctoral nursing students, maternal-child health nurses and social workers, nurse midwives, medical students, obstetricians, pediatricians, legislators, and policy makers. The book also should be of interest to women's studies and feminist scholars, and to the general public, especially childbearing women.

We are indebted to our study participants. Those women, who gave so much of their time and shared so much of their lives, made this study possible. We also are indebted to our research assistants, Trish Dunphy, Mary Beth Haas, Kathleen Higgins, Bonnie Mauger Graff, Denise Fair, Barbara Koch, Patricia Rollo, Gail Staudt, and Jean Whelan, without whose help we could not have enrolled all of the study participants and conducted all of the home visits to collect the data. Furthermore, we are indebted to Judith Wojechowski Smith, who provided secretarial support and transcribed the audiotapes of our interviews with the women.

Lorraine Tulman
Jacqueline Fawcett

Part I

INTRODUCTION

1

A Theory of Adaptation
During Childbearing

Pregnancy and the postpartum are times of considerable transition in the life of a woman. Previous research has focused on the process of maternal role attainment and factors influencing transition to the maternal role (Mercer, 1986, 1995; Rubin, 1984). Other, now classic studies have explored the extent to which achievement of parenthood is regarded as a crisis (Hobbs, 1965; Hobbs & Cole, 1976) and examined psychological responses to childbearing (Ahmed, 1981; Blum, 1980; Colman & Colman, 1971; Grossman et al., 1980; Shereshefsky & Yarrow, 1973). Moreover, textbook descriptions of the postpartum continue to focus primarily on healing of reproductive organs and the taking on of the maternal role during the first few weeks after delivery (Cunningham, MacDonald, & Gant, 1997; Reeder, Martin, & Koniak-Griffin, 1997). Thus, little is known of the social response to pregnancy and the postpartum in the form of alterations in the woman's general health. More important, existing legislation regulating maternity leave reflects a sick role definition of medical disability and the presence of medical complications rather than a broader health definition including usual role performance (Pregnancy Discrimination Act of 1978; Family and Medical Leave Act of 1993).

Given that more than half of married women with children less than one year of age have been part of the labor force for many years (Bachu & O'Connell, 2001), our study of women's health during pregnancy and following childbirth has potentially important clinical and socioeconomic implications. Indeed, enhanced knowledge of alterations in women's health during pregnancy and the postpartum provides an empirical base for formulating clinical interventions to improve health during pregnancy and the postpartum, as well as a data-based social policy regarding maternity leave.

Although childbearing typically is characterized as a period of good health for most women in the United States, medical and nursing textbooks describe the time after delivery as one of recovery from childbearing, thereby implying that pregnancy and delivery are illnesses.

3

We believe that adaptation is a more accurate perspective and, therefore, we view both pregnancy and the postpartum as times of considerable and often profound change to which each woman adapts. In this book, we report the results of our longitudinal study of women's health during pregnancy and the postpartum—including physical and psychosocial health, functional status, and family relationships.

We present the framework for our study in this chapter. We designed the study to test our Theory of Adaptation During Childbearing, which was derived from the Roy Adaptation Model (Figure 1.1), a conceptual model of nursing. In this chapter, we first present an overview of the Roy Adaptation Model and then describe our Theory of Adaptation During Childbearing. For the reader who would like more detail, we have provided the definitions of study variables, a description of the study sample and the instruments, including psychometric properties and scoring procedures, and a description of the data collection procedures in the Appendix.

Inasmuch as we began planning and designing the study in the late 1980s, we used as a guide the Roy Adaptation Model as presented in Roy's 1984 book, *Introduction to Nursing: An Adaptation Model* (2nd ed.), and in Andrews and Roy's 1986 book, *Essentials of the Roy Adaptation Model.*

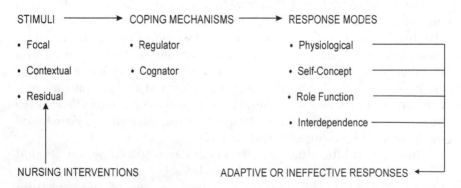

ROY ADAPTATION MODEL

ADAPTIVE SYSTEM

STIMULI ⟶ COPING MECHANISMS ⟶ RESPONSE MODES

- Focal   - Regulator   - Physiological
- Contextual   - Cognator   - Self-Concept
- Residual   - Role Function
                                      - Interdependence

NURSING INTERVENTIONS   ADAPTIVE OR INEFFECTIVE RESPONSES ⟵

FIGURE 1.1   Diagram of the Roy Adaptation Model.

THE ROY ADAPTATION MODEL

The Roy Adaptation Model depicts the individual as a human *adaptive system* who interacts with constantly changing focal, contextual, and residual stimuli that arise in the environment. The *focal stimulus* is the one most immediately confronting the person. The *contextual stimuli* are all other stimuli that contribute directly to adaptation. The *residual stimuli* are other unknown factors that may influence the situation; when the factors making up residual stimuli become known, they usually are considered contextual stimuli, but also may be focal stimuli.

Individuals respond to environmental stimuli through regulator and cognator coping mechanisms. The *regulator coping mechanism* encompasses basic neural, chemical, and endocrine channels that process stimuli in an automatic, unconscious manner. The *cognator coping mechanism* encompasses four cognitive-emotive channels for stimulus processing: perceptual/information processing, learning, judgment, and emotion.

Regulator and cognator processes are manifested in four response modes. The *physiological mode* emphasizes maintenance of the physiological integrity of the adaptive system. The *self-concept mode* focuses on psychic integrity and deals with perception of the physical self and the personal self. The *role function mode* deals with social integrity by focusing on performance of activities associated with the various roles one enacts throughout life. The *interdependence mode* also deals with social integrity and emphasizes behaviors underlying the development and maintenance of satisfying affectional relationships with significant others, as well as the provision and receipt of social support.

Responses are classified as adaptive or ineffective. *Adaptive responses* are those that meet the human adaptive system's goals for survival, growth, reproduction, and mastery. *Ineffective responses* are those that do not meet those goals and, therefore, signal a need for intervention.

Nursing intervention involves the management of environmental stimuli. Management encompasses increasing, decreasing, maintaining, removing, or otherwise altering or changing relevant focal and/or contextual stimuli.

DERIVATION OF THE THEORY OF ADAPTATION DURING CHILDBEARING

We derived our Theory of Adaptation During Childbearing from the following concepts of the Roy Adaptation Model: *adaptive system, focal stimulus, contextual stimuli, physiological mode, self-concept mode, role function mode,* and *interdependence mode.* We linked each conceptual model concept with a component, or concept, of our Theory of Adaptation During Childbearing. We then used an assortment of questionnaires and an interview schedule to measure the theory concepts. A diagram depicting the linkages between the Roy Adaptation Model concepts, the theory concepts, and their measurements is displayed in Figure 1.2.

The *adaptive system* of interest in our theory was the childbearing woman. We enrolled 250 initially low-risk women in the study. Between recruitment and delivery, 12 women voluntarily withdrew and 5 women spontaneously aborted. In addition, third trimester data were not collected from five of the six women who delivered prematurely and one woman who was not able to be scheduled for a third trimester visit before she delivered. Our pregnancy sample, therefore, was made up of the 227 women who provided us with complete data for all three trimesters.

After delivery, an additional three women voluntarily withdrew from our study, one woman's infant died at four months of a rare genetic disease, and three additional women were pregnant again by six months postpartum and, therefore, were not included in the analysis of the postpartum data. Our postpartum data did, however, include the 6 women who did not provide third trimester data, yielding a total postpartum sample of 226 women.

The women who participated in our study ranged in age from 19 to 41 years. All had completed high school and more than two thirds were college graduates. Approximately three quarters of the women were employed at the time of recruitment, and more than one half were employed at six months after delivery. The vast majority (93%) of the women were White; 4% were African American; 2%, Asian; and 1%, Hispanic. Eighty-two percent had vaginal deliveries. Thirty-nine percent delivered their first child; 44%, their second; and 17%, their third, fourth, fifth, or sixth child.

The *focal stimulus* was represented in our theory by pregnancy and the postpartum, which were operationalized by collecting data from the women at the end of each trimester of pregnancy (at 12 to 14 weeks, 25 to 27 weeks, and 36 to 37 weeks of gestation) and at 3 weeks, 6 weeks, 3 months, and 6 months after delivery.

The *contextual stimuli* were represented in our theory by maternal demographic characteristics, specifically maternal age, education, occupation, and employment status; place of residence; household composi-

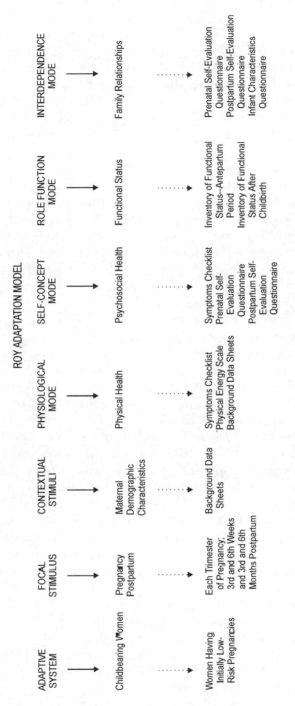

FIGURE 1.2 Linkages between the Roy Adaptation Model, the Theory of Adaptation During Childbearing, and study measures.

tion; household income; maternity leave and compensation policies of the employer; and job income lost due to childbearing. Items on the *Background Data Sheets* measured all of those characteristics.

The *physiological mode* was represented in our theory by physical health. Data were collected from the participants on physical symptoms; physical energy; prepregnancy weight, weight gain during pregnancy, postpartum weight, postpartum weight loss, and postpartum weight retention; parity; minor prenatal, intrapartal, postpartal, and neonatal complications; type of delivery; medical restrictions on activities; and method of infant feeding. Physical symptoms were measured by the *Symptoms Checklist* (Fawcett & York, 1986). Physical energy was measured by the investigator-developed *Physical Energy Scale*. Body weight and height were measured by the women's self-report and recorded on the *Background Data Sheets*. All other physical health variables were measured by data obtained in interviews with the participating women and recorded on the *Background Data Sheets*.

The *self-concept mode* was represented in our theory by psychosocial health. The study variables were psychological symptoms; acceptance of pregnancy; identification of a motherhood role; preparation for labor; fear of pain, helplessness, and loss of control during labor; concern for well-being of self and baby; gratification with labor and delivery; life satisfaction; satisfaction with motherhood; and maternal confidence in ability to cope with tasks of motherhood. Psychological symptoms were measured by the *Symptoms Checklist* (Fawcett & York, 1986). Acceptance of pregnancy; identification of a motherhood role; preparation for labor; fear of pain, helplessness, and loss of control during labor; and concern for well-being of self and baby were measured by scales on the *Prenatal Self-Evaluation Questionnaire* (Lederman, 1984, 1996; Lederman, Lederman, Work, & McCann, 1979). Gratification with labor and delivery, life satisfaction, satisfaction with the parental role, and maternal confidence in ability to cope with tasks of motherhood were measured by scales on the *Postpartum Self-Evaluation Questionnaire* (Lederman, Weingarten, & Lederman, 1981).

The *role function mode* was represented in our theory by functional status. Functional status during pregnancy was measured by the *Inventory of Functional Status-Antepartum Period* (Tulman et al., 1991). Postpartum functional status was measured by the *Inventory of Functional Status After Childbirth* (Fawcett, Tulman, & Myers, 1988).

The *interdependence mode* was represented in our theory by family relationships. The study variables were the woman's relationship with her own mother, relationship with husband during pregnancy, social support from family and friends, quality of the marital relationship after delivery, maternal perception of father's participation in child care, maternal perception of infant temperament, and infant nocturnal sleep. The woman's relationship with her own mother and relationship with husband during pregnancy were measured by scales on the *Prenatal Self-Evaluation Questionnaire* (Lederman, 1984, 1996; Lederman et al., 1979). Social support from family and friends, quality of the marital relationship after delivery, and maternal perception of father's participation in child care were measured by scales on the *Postpartum Self-Evaluation Questionnaire* (Lederman, Weingarten, & Lederman, 1981). Maternal perception of infant temperament was measured by the *Infant Characteristics Questionnaire* (Bates, Freeland, & Lounsbury, 1979). Infant nocturnal sleep was measured by an item on the *Background Data Sheets.*

We selected two propositions from the Roy Adaptation Model to guide the development of the propositions of our Theory of Adaptation During Childbearing. First, the Roy Adaptation Model proposes that changes in stimuli are associated with changes in responses. We therefore proposed that physical health, psychosocial health, functional status, and family relationships would change as the pregnancy and the postpartum progressed (Figure 1.3 [A]).

Second, the Roy Adaptation Model proposes that the response modes are interrelated, such that responses in any one mode have an effect on, or act as a stimulus for, one or all of the other modes. Thus, we proposed that physical health and functional status, psychosocial health and functional status, and family relationships and functional status would be related (Figure 1.3 [B, C, D]).

In summary, we derived our Theory of Adaptation During Childbearing from selected concepts and propositions of the Roy Adaptation Model. Our theory proposes that physical health, psychosocial health, functional status, and family relationships change during pregnancy and the postpartum. The theory further proposes that physical health, psychosocial health, and family relationships are related to functional status during pregnancy and the postpartum. We designed our longitudinal study specifically to test the theory. The results of our study and our conclusions about our findings are presented in Parts II, III, and IV of this book.

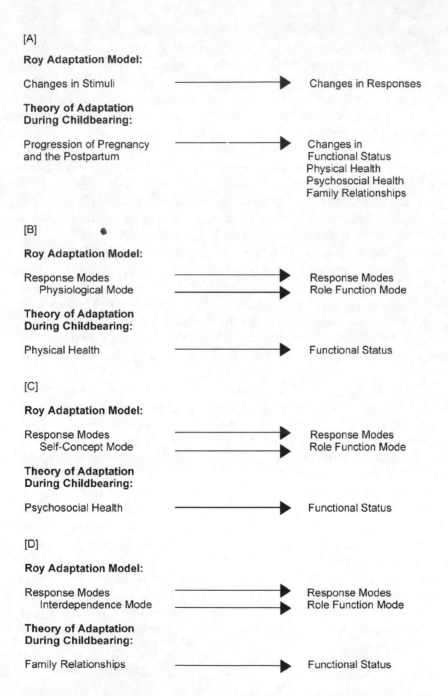

[A]

Roy Adaptation Model:

Changes in Stimuli ⟶ Changes in Responses

**Theory of Adaptation
During Childbearing:**

Progression of Pregnancy ⟶ Changes in
and the Postpartum Functional Status
Physical Health
Psychosocial Health
Family Relationships

[B]

Roy Adaptation Model:

Response Modes ⟶ Response Modes
Physiological Mode ⟶ Role Function Mode

**Theory of Adaptation
During Childbearing:**

Physical Health ⟶ Functional Status

[C]

Roy Adaptation Model:

Response Modes ⟶ Response Modes
Self-Concept Mode ⟶ Role Function Mode

**Theory of Adaptation
During Childbearing:**

Psychosocial Health ⟶ Functional Status

[D]

Roy Adaptation Model:

Response Modes ⟶ Response Modes
Interdependence Mode ⟶ Role Function Mode

**Theory of Adaptation
During Childbearing:**

Family Relationships ⟶ Functional Status

FIGURE 1.3 Diagrams of conceptual model and theory propositions.

REFERENCES

Ahmed, P. (Ed.) (1981). *Pregnancy, childbirth, and parenthood.* New York: Elsevier.

Andrews, H. A., & Roy, C. (1986). *Essentials of the Roy Adaptation Model.* Norwalk, CT: Appleton-Century-Crofts.

Bachu, A., & O'Connell, M. (2001). Fertility of American women: June 2000. *Current Population Reports, P20–543RV.* Washington, DC: U.S. Census Bureau.

Bates, J. E., Freeland, C. A., & Lounsbury, M. L. (1979). Measurement of infant difficultness. *Child Development, 50,* 794–803.

Blum, B. L. (Ed.) (1980). *Psychological aspects of pregnancy, birthing, and bonding.* New York: Human Sciences Press.

Colman, A. D., & Colman, L. L. (1971). *Pregnancy: The psychological experience.* New York: Herder and Herder.

Cunningham, F. G., MacDonald, P. C., & Gant, N. F. (1997). *William's obstetrics* (20th ed.). Stamford, CT: Appleton & Lange.

Fawcett, J., Tulman, L., & Myers, S. T. (1988). Development of the Inventory of Functional Status after Childbirth. *Journal of Nurse-Midwifery, 33,* 252–260.

Fawcett, J., & York, R. (1986). Spouses' physical and psychological symptoms during pregnancy and the postpartum. *Nursing Research, 35,* 144–148.

Grossman, F. K., Eichler, L. S., Winickoff, S. A., Anzalone, M. K., Gofseyeff, M. H., & Sargent, S. P. (1980). *Pregnancy, birth, and parenthood.* San Francisco: Jossey-Bass.

Hobbs, D. F. (1965). Parenthood as crisis: A third study. *Journal of Marriage and the Family, 27,* 367–378.

Hobbs, D. F., & Cole, S. P. (1976). Transition to parenthood: A decade of replications. *Journal of Marriage and the Family, 38,* 723–731.

Lederman, R. P. (1984). *Psychosocial adaptation in pregnancy: Assessment of seven dimensions of maternal development.* Englewood Cliffs, NJ: Prentice-Hall.

Lederman, R. P. (1996). *Psychosocial adaptation in pregnancy: Assessment of seven dimensions of maternal development* (2nd ed.). New York: Springer Publishing.

Lederman, R. P., Lederman, E., Work, B. A., Jr., & McCann, D. S. (1979). Relationship of psychological factors in pregnancy to progress in labor. *Nursing Research, 28,* 94–97.

Lederman, R. P., Weingarten, C. G., & Lederman, E. (1981). Postpartum Self-Evaluation Questionnaire: Measure of maternal adaptation. In R. P. Lederman, B. S. Raff, & P. Carroll (Eds.), *Perinatal parental behavior: Nursing research and implications* (Birth Defects: Original Article Series, Vol. 17, No. 6, pp. 201–231). New York: Alan R. Liss.

Mercer, R. T. (1986). *First-time motherhood.* New York: Springer Publishing.

Mercer, R. T. (1995). *Becoming a mother: Research on maternal identity from Rubin to the present.* New York: Springer Publishing.

Reeder, S. J., Martin, L. L., & Koniak-Griffin, D. (1997). *Maternity nursing. Family, newborn, and women's health care* (18th ed.). Philadelphia: Lippincott-Raven.

Rubin, R. (1984). *Maternal identity and the maternal experience.* New York: Springer Publishing.

Roy, C. (1984). *Introduction to nursing: An adaptation model* (2nd ed.). Englewood Cliffs, NJ: Prentice-Hall.

Shereshefsky, P. M., & Yarrow, L. J. (1973). *Psychological aspects of a first pregnancy and early postnatal adaptation.* New York: Raven Press.

Tulman, L., Higgins, K., Fawcett, J., Nunno, C., Vansickel, C., Haas, M. B., & Speca, M. M. (1991). The Inventory of Functional Status-Antepartum Period: Development and testing. *Journal of Nurse-Midwifery, 36,* 117–123.

Part II

ADAPTATION DURING PREGNANCY

2

Physical Health and Functional Status During Pregnancy

Women's health during pregnancy has been studied primarily in terms of occurrences of obstetrical complications and worsening of pre-existing chronic illnesses (Cunningham, MacDonald, & Gant, 1997). Little is known, however, about the more subtle changes experienced by low-risk pregnant women as they adapt during childbearing. In particular, no other investigators have, to date, tracked changes in physical energy, physical symptoms, and functional status, or closely examined the relations of physical energy and physical symptoms to functional status during the three trimesters of pregnancy. In this chapter, we present the part of our Theory of Adaptation During Childbearing that deals with functional status and two physical health variables—physical energy and physical symptoms—during pregnancy (Figures 2.1 and 2.2). In keeping with the Roy Adaptation Model and the available evidence from the literature, we proposed that functional status, physical energy, and physical symptoms would change from the first to the second to the third trimester of pregnancy (Figure 2.2 [A]). We also proposed that physical energy and physical symptoms would be related to functional status during each trimester of pregnancy (Figure 2.2 [B]).

ROLE THEORY AND FUNCTIONAL STATUS

Although some attention in the literature has been given to the process of, and factors influencing, attainment of the role of mother, little attention has been given to how childbearing influences the performance of other roles. In keeping with the Roy Adaptation Model (Roy, 1984), our conceptualization and definition of functional status is based on tenets of classical role theory. We view functional status as the action component of roles, that is, the performance of behaviors associated with roles. Drawing from the work of Goffman (1961) and Parsons and Shils (1951), Nuwayhid (1984) noted that role refers to the title given to the individual, as well as to the behaviors expected to be performed

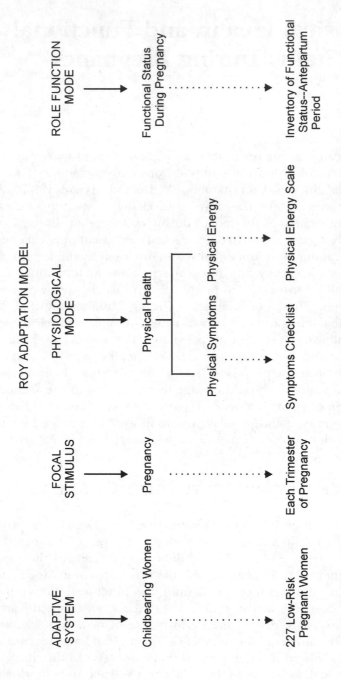

FIGURE 2.1 Linkages between the Roy Adaptation Model, physical health and functional status, and study variables and measures.

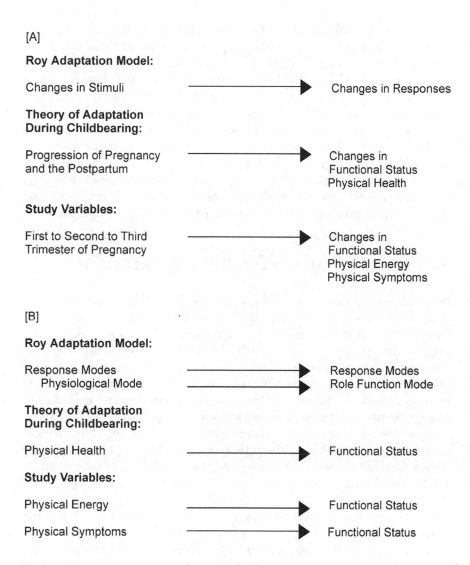

FIGURE 2.2 Diagrams of propositions of the Roy Adaptation Model, the Theory of Adaptation During Childbearing, and study variables: Functional status and physical health during pregnancy.

to maintain the title. Role performance, in turn, is "the collection of behaviors observed when an individual with a particular title undertakes those actions that society attributes to a person with that title" (Nuwayhid, 1984, p. 286). Turner (1978), a renowned role theorist, indicated that role-taking is a reciprocal process, such that each new role requires adjustments in the behaviors associated with existing roles. Turner's work suggests that changes should occur in the performance of various established roles during the childbearing period, when the maternal role is being attained. Accordingly, we have defined functional status during pregnancy as the extent to which the pregnant woman continues her usual role activities, including personal care, household, social and community, child care, occupational, and educational activities.

FUNCTIONAL STATUS DURING PREGNANCY

Pregnancy requires changes in social interactions and lifestyle, including daily routines and priorities placed on various activities (Campbell & Field, 1989). Indeed, our own and colleagues' clinical observations suggest that childbearing women's alterations in role activities begin during pregnancy. Research findings provide more systematic evidence of alternations in role activities. As we were developing the *Inventory of Functional Status—Antepartum Period*, we found preliminary evidence of changes in pregnant women's performance of usual activities. The pregnant women in our sample commented that they could no longer perform certain activities without help, such as cleaning house, washing dishes, doing laundry, and caring for their children (Tulman et al., 1991). Bungum and colleagues (2000) reported that just 44 (32%) of the 137 women in their study engaged in active exercise during the first and second trimesters of pregnancy; a large majority (79%) of the women who exercised during pregnancy also had engaged in active exercise prior to the pregnancy. Imle (1990) found that during the third trimester, women were concerned about changes in their daily routines, which is an aspect of functional status. Schramm, Stockbauer, and Hoffman (1996) reported that 79% of the women in their study stopped working, and just 16% continued to exercise during the third trimester.

Ales and Norton (1989) found evidence of a progressive deterioration in physical function as pregnancy progressed, which was accompanied by a decrease in the percentage of women who worked outside the home from the second trimester (62%) to the third trimester (33%). Wildschut, Harker, and Riddoch (1993), however, found no association between length of gestation and report of hard physical activity or exercise in a sample of 100 mostly first and second trimester pregnant British women.

PHYSICAL HEALTH DURING PREGNANCY

Andrews and Roy (1986) postulated that role performance is influenced by physical health, but little attention has been given to identification of specific variables that are related to the performance of existing roles during pregnancy. We selected two physical health variables—physical energy and physical symptoms.

Physical Energy

Pregnancy takes a toll on the woman's physical energy. Hall (1991) reported that women experience an overall lack of energy during pregnancy. Kelley and Boyle (1995) found that all 10 of the women who participated in their qualitative study experienced a diminished level of energy during the pregnancy. Condon (1987) provided more precise data; he found that almost one quarter (24%) of the 101 women in his cross-sectional study reported a severe to very severe lack of energy at some time during the pregnancy.

   Physical energy is conceptually related to energy expenditure (Piers et al., 1995) and fatigue (Lee & DeJoseph, 1992; Milligan & Pugh, 1994; Pugh & Milligan, 1993; Reeves, Potempa, & Gallo, 1991; van Lier, Manteuffel, DiIorio, & Stalcup, 1993). Although overlaps in these variables seem intuitive, definitions and research findings indicate some distinctions. For example, Pugh and Milligan's (1993) definition of fatigue during childbearing extends beyond energy level. Furthermore, Lee and colleagues (1994) differentiated between energy and fatigue in their assessment of a sample of nonpregnant women, and found a very low correlation between scores for vitality, which included items about energy level, and a fatigue severity score. In addition, Lee, Hicks, and Nino-Murcia's (1991) visual analog scale, which they designed to measure fatigue, included separate subscales for level of fatigue and level of energy.

Studies of perceived fatigue have revealed differences between pregnant and nonpregnant women, as well as changes during pregnancy.
Behrenz and Monga (1999) reported that first trimester pregnant
women experienced greater fatigue and spent more time sleeping than
their nonpregnant counterparts. Pugh and Milligan (1995) found that
fatigue increased from the first to the second trimester and from the
second to the third trimester in a pilot study of 11 women. Lee and
Zaffke (1999) found that their sample of 30 women reported that level
of fatigue changed during pregnancy, with the lowest level during the
second trimester and the highest level during the third trimester. More
relevant to our study are Condon's (1987) and Lee and Zaffke's (1999)
findings that women reported changes in level of energy during each
trimester of pregnancy, with a higher level occurring in the second
trimester than in the first or third trimesters.

Physical Energy and Functional Status

No studies of the relation between energy level and overall functional
status during pregnancy were located. Instead, research has focused on
components of functional status and fatigue. Brown (1987) found that
fatigue was greater in pregnant women who were employed than in
their unemployed counterparts. In addition, Reeves and colleagues
(1991) reported that fatigue had a substantial impact on women's performance of household and social activities during the first half of
pregnancy.

Physical Symptoms

Narrative descriptions of pregnancy typically include mention of the
"common complaints" or "minor discomforts" of the childbearing period (Cunningham, McDonald, & Gant, 1997; Davis, 1996; Reeder,
Martin, & Koniak-Griffin, 1997), and researchers have begun to system-
atically document the type and frequency of such physical symptoms
during pregnancy. Hall's (1991) analysis of interview data revealed that
women experienced fluid gain, cramps, backache, and nausea during
pregnancy. Mindell and Jacobson (2000) found that many women experience sleep disturbances throughout pregnancy, including frequent
night wakings, difficulty falling asleep, and symptoms of sleep apnea.

Condon (1987) reported that in a sample of 101 pregnant women, almost 34% experienced sleep disturbances, 11% experienced appetite disturbances, 25% experienced aches and pains, and 6% experienced nausea/vomiting, all of which they rated as severe to very severe at some time during the pregnancy.

The available empirical evidence indicates that some changes occur in the number and type of physical symptoms experienced during each trimester of pregnancy. Lips (1985) found that women experienced different clusters of physical symptoms during each trimester of pregnancy. The first trimester was characterized by nausea/vomiting, dizziness/fainting, backache, general aches and pains, and heaviness. The second trimester was characterized by backache, general aches and pains, and heaviness. The third trimester was characterized by swelling, backache, general aches and pains, heaviness, and feeling uncomfortable. Fawcett and York (1986) found that the most frequent physical symptoms reported by a group of 23 women were feeling tired, increased urination, being less active than usual, feeling bloated, increased appetite, sensitivity to odors, and nausea and/or vomiting during the third to fourth month of pregnancy. In the ninth month of pregnancy, the most frequent symptoms reported by a group of 24 women were feeling tired, increased urination, indigestion, backache, being less active than usual, feeling clumsy or awkward, nausea and/or vomiting, increased appetite, sensitivity to odors, and difficulty breathing (Fawcett & York, 1986). Drake, Verhulst, and Fawcett (1988) reported a similar list of physical symptoms for 20 pregnant women, but did not distinguish symptoms by trimester. Gulick, Shaw, and Allison (1989) reported that at least some of the 50 African-American pregnant women in their study experienced nausea, vomiting, tiredness, headache, difficulty sleeping, heartburn, constipation, and general discomfort during the first or third trimester. Mindell and Jacobson (2000) found that 45% of the 38 third trimester women in their study reported taking daytime naps, and 97% reported waking during the night.

Lerum and LoBiondo-Wood (1989) found that a sample of 80 low-risk second trimester pregnant women experienced a variety of physical symptoms often and rated those symptoms as moderate to severe. They did not, however, provide a list of the symptoms. Gjerdingen, Froberg, and Kochevar (1991) found evidence of few physical symptoms among a group of 37 women who were more than 20 weeks pregnant but again, did not provide a list of the symptoms.

Back pain is experienced by approximately one half of all pregnant women (Colliton, 1996; Kristiansson, Svardsudd, & von Schoultz, 1996;

Östgaard, Andersson, & Karlsson, 1991; Östgaard, Zetherström, Roos-Hansson, & Svanberg, 1994), with pain in the sacroiliac area increasing during pregnancy. Although he did not specify the source, Condon (1987) reported that pregnant women experienced more aches and pains during the third trimester than during the first or second trimesters. Moreover, investigators have found that nausea and vomiting occur more frequently and with greater severity during pregnancy than is generally believed (Hyde, 1989; O'Brien & Naber, 1992; O'Brien, Relyea, & Taerum, 1996), especially during the first trimester (Condon, 1987; Gulick, Shaw, & Allison, 1989). DiIorio, van Lier, and Manteuffel (1992) reported that first trimester nausea and vomiting were prevalent between 3 p.m. and 6 p.m., a time when most women were at work; they postulated that the timing of the occurrence of these symptoms altered the women's lifestyle.

Physical Symptoms and Functional Status

The literature supports a relation between physical symptoms and functional status during pregnancy. In general, good physical health during the childbearing period is associated with a higher level of functional status, in the forms of work productivity and parental competence, than poor health (Brown, 1989). Fast and colleagues (1990) found that back pain interfered with activities of daily living for about 10% of pregnant women. Brown (1987) reported that homemakers experienced more backaches during the second and third trimesters of pregnancy than their employed counterparts. Horns and colleagues (1995) found that women who exercised actively during the third trimester of pregnancy had fewer physical symptoms than their sedentary counterparts.

THE RESULTS OF OUR STUDY

We examined our data from the 227 women who participated in our study throughout pregnancy for changes in overall and specific areas of functional status, and in physical energy and physical symptoms (Table 2.1). In addition, we looked at the correlations between physical energy and functional status and physical symptoms and functional status (Table 2.2). We also explored the women's responses to our interviews with them at six months postpartum, when we asked them

TABLE 2.1   Functional Status, Physical Energy, and Physical Symptoms During Pregnancy

Variable	First Trimester	Second Trimester	Third Trimester	p
FUNCTIONAL STATUS [M, SD]**				
Household ($n = 227$)	2.49 (.42)	2.60 (.31)	2.36 (.42)	< .0005[b]
Social/Community ($n = 225$)	2.58 (.48)	2.56 (.46)	2.36 (.52)	< .0005[a]
Child Care ($n = 144$)	2.73 (.33)	2.71 (.29)	2.56 (.38)	< .0005[a]
Personal Care ($n = 226$)	2.33 (.60)	2.45 (.51)	2.20 (.55)	< .0005[b]
Occupational ($n = 109$)	2.62 (.56)	2.79 (.39)	2.56 (.56)	< .0005[b]
Educational ($n = 11$)	2.50 (.67)	2.47 (.79)	2.52 (.46)	.93
Total ($N = 227$)	2.55 (.37)	2.63 (.27)	2.39 (.38)	< .0005[b]
MAINTAIN USUAL LEVEL OF PHYSICAL ENERGY [%]				< .00005[b]
Not At All	27%	9%	26%	
Partially	61%	57%	59%	
Fully	12%	34%	15%	
NUMBER OF PHYSICAL SYMPTOMS [M, SD]*	8.82 (2.67)	8.82 (3.10)	9.71 (2.86)	< .0005[a]

[a]Difference between second trimester and third trimester statistically significant.
[b]Differences between first trimester and second trimester and second trimester and third trimester statistically significant.
*Potential range of scores = 0–21 symptoms.
**Potential range of scores = 1.00–3.00; higher scores indicate greater functional status.

TABLE 2.2   Correlations of Physical Energy and Physical Symptoms With Functional Status During Pregnancy ($N = 227$)

Variable	First Trimester Functional Status	Second Trimester Functional Status	Third Trimester Functional Status
PHYSICAL ENERGY	.448**	.311**	.348**
PHYSICAL SYMPTOMS	−.260**	−.294**	−.156*

*$p < .05$
**$p < .0005$

to reflect on their experiences during pregnancy. They told us a great deal about how their level of energy and physical symptoms helped them or hindered them in their attempts to continue their usual activities during pregnancy.

Changes in Functional Status

Overall functional status and functional status in the specific areas of household, personal care, and occupational activities changed during pregnancy ($p < .0005$), with an increase from the first to the second trimester, and then a decrease during the third trimester (Table 2.1). Functional status in social and community activities and child care activities also changed during pregnancy ($p < .0005$). For these activities, no changes were found from the first to second trimester, but there was a decrease between the second and third trimesters. In addition, just 11 of the women were involved in educational activities during pregnancy; no evidence of a change in functional status in these activities was found.

We then divided the women's overall functional status scores into two categories—less than full functional status and full functional status. The percentage of women reporting full functional status differed by trimester of pregnancy ($p < .00005$), with an increase from the first (62%) to the second trimester (70%), and a decrease from the second to the third (47%) trimester.

Changes in Physical Energy

The women's level of physical energy changed over the course of pregnancy ($p < .00005$), with an increase from the first to the second trimester of pregnancy, and then a decrease from the second to the third trimester (Table 2.1). Relatively few women reported maintaining their usual prepregnant level of physical energy during pregnancy—just 12% during the first trimester, 34% during the second trimester, and 15% during the third trimester.

Physical Energy and Functional Status

The correlations between physical energy and functional status were of moderate magnitude (Table 2.2). The positive correlation between physical energy and functional status was statistically significant during each trimester of pregnancy ($p < .0005$). Thus, women who fully maintained their usual level of physical energy also performed their usual activities at a higher level than did the women who did not maintain or only partially maintained their usual level of physical energy.

More than one quarter (28%) of the women told us, when interviewed at six months postpartum, that they continued their usual activities during pregnancy because they had sufficient energy or were able to conserve energy by taking naps or sleeping more than usual. One women stated that she had "More energy than usual." Another woman explained, "If I could get a nap during the day, that helped me do what I had to do. If I could get a little extra sleep, I had the energy to do what I had to do." Paradoxically, another woman commented, "I learned how to function on a very low level of energy."

Conversely, almost two fifths (39%) of the women indicated that they were hindered in the performance of their usual activities by a lack of energy or feeling tired. One woman stated, "I expected to have more energy than I had by the end." Other women's comments implied that their feelings of tiredness were related to their level of energy. One woman, for example, stated that she was hindered by "feeling tired, mostly in the afternoon." Another woman said, "I got tired very easily." Still another woman commented, "I was not able to keep up [due to] tiredness." And another explained, "I wasn't hindered until the eighth month, [when] I was very tired and it was hard to stand on my feet."

Changes in Physical Symptoms

The number of physical symptoms experienced by the women remained unchanged from the first to the second trimester of pregnancy, but increased from the second and third trimester ($p < .0005$) (Table 2.1). The most common physical symptoms during the first trimester, in decreasing order of frequency, were feeling tired, nausea and vomiting, increased urination, decreased activity, and sensitivity to odors. During the second trimester, the most common physical symptoms were increased urination, feeling tired, backache, increased appetite, and heartburn. During the third trimester, the most common physical symptoms were increased urination, feeling tired, feeling warmer than usual, decreased activity, and heartburn.

Physical Symptoms and Functional Status

There was a statistically significant negative correlation between the number of physical symptoms and functional status during each trimester ($p < .05$). That is, regardless of the trimester of pregnancy, as the number of physical symptoms increased, the women's overall performance of their usual activities decreased. These correlations were, however, of low magnitude (Table 2.2).

More than one quarter (27%) of the women told us that they were hindered in the performance of their usual activities by various physical symptoms. One woman explained that she experienced "heartburn, hemorrhoids, bloating of my lower extremities, that sort of thing. I would say that hindered my usual activities." Another woman commented that she was hindered by "some of the bad symptoms, like morning, noon, and night sickness up until five months." Still another women noted that she was hindered by "sickness, including nausea and vomiting, extreme fatigue, [and] aches and pains." A woman who experienced back pain stated, "There [were] some days I could not move." In contrast, a few (2%) women indicated that a lack of physical symptoms helped them to continue their usual activities.

CONCLUSION

Women's physical health and functional status changed over the three trimesters of pregnancy. As expected from our Theory of Adaptation During Childbearing and in keeping with the Roy Adaptation Model, changes occurred in the variables representing the physiological and role function modes as the focal stimulus of pregnancy progressed. Moreover, the correlations between the variables representing the Roy Adaptation Model physiological and role function response modes indicate that these modes are interrelated components of adaptation during pregnancy. The finding of relations between those two Roy Adaptation Model response modes lends additional support to the results of a meta-analysis that examined the interrelations between the modes (Chiou, 2000).

Our finding of changes in functional status during the three trimesters of pregnancy contrasts with Wildschut and colleagues' (1993) finding of no association between length of gestation and activity. Our finding that women experienced greatest functional status during the second trimester is consistent with textbook descriptions of feelings of maximal well-being at that time (Pillitteri, 1998). Our finding of lowest functional status toward the end of the third trimester also is consistent with textbook descriptions of overall feelings as pregnancy comes to an end (Pillitteri, 1998), as well as with Schramm and colleagues' (1996) finding of less activity during the third trimester. Indeed, more than one-half (53%) of the women in our study reported that they were at less than full functional status during the third trimester.

Our finding of changes in the level of physical energy during the three trimesters of pregnancy is similar to Pugh and Milligan's (1995) pilot study data. Our finding of no change in the number of physical symptoms from the first to the second trimester of pregnancy conflicts with McRae's (1990) finding of a slight decrease in physical symptoms during the second trimester, followed by a return to the first trimester level during the third trimester. McRae, however, collected data only during the second trimester and at 12 weeks postpartum. Thus, she relied on recall for measurement of first and third trimester physical symptoms.

Our finding of an increase in the number of physical symptoms from the second to the third trimester of pregnancy conflicts with Brown's (1988) finding of no changes during those two trimesters. Brown's study was cross-sectional in design, however, and the sample was limited to women in the late second trimester (16%) and the third trimester (84%). Furthermore, the women were asked to retrospectively report the occurrence of symptoms since the beginning of pregnancy.

Taken together, our findings of a positive correlation between physical energy and functional status and a negative correlation between physical symptoms and functional status during pregnancy suggest that the level of energy and number of symptoms may have affected the women's ability to perform usual activities (i.e., functional ability), which in turn affected their actual performance of activities (i.e., functional status). This distinction between functional ability and functional status is consistent with thinking about the dimensions of functioning and their interrelations (Richmond, McCorkle, Tulman, & Fawcett, 1997). This line of reasoning also is consistent with Ales and Norton's (1989) finding of a negative relation between ability to perform activities and employment status. Additional research is recommended to determine whether a sequential relation exists from physical symptoms to physical energy to functional ability to functional status.

REFERENCES

Ales, K. L., & Norton, M. E. (1989). Changes in functional status during pregnancy. *American Journal of the Medical Sciences, 297,* 355–360.

Andrews, H. A., & Roy, C. (1986). *Essentials of the Roy Adaptation Model.* Norwalk, CT: Appleton-Century-Crofts.

Behrenz, K. M., & Monga, M. (1999). Fatigue in pregnancy: A comparative study. *American Journal of Perinatology, 16,* 185–188.

Brown, M. A. (1987). Employment during pregnancy: Influences on women's health and social support. *Health Care for Women International, 8,* 151–167.

Brown, M. A. (1988). A comparison of health responses in expectant mothers and fathers. *Western Journal of Nursing Research, 10,* 527–549.

Brown, M. A. (1989). *Expectant parents' perceptions of their work productivity.* Paper presented at meeting of American Nurses' Association Council of Nurse Researchers, Chicago, Illinois.

Bungum, T. J., Peaslee, D. L., Jackson, A. W., & Perez, M. A. (2000). Exercise during pregnancy and type of delivery in nulliparae. *Journal of Obstetric, Gynecologic, and Neonatal Nursing, 29,* 258–264.

Campbell, I. E., & Field, P. A. (1989). Common psychological concerns experienced by parents during pregnancy. *Canada's Mental Health, 37*(1), 2–5.

Chiou, C-P. (2000). A meta-analysis of the interrelationships between the modes in Roy's Adaptation Model. *Nursing Science Quarterly, 13,* 252–258.

Colliton, J. (1996). Back pain and pregnancy: Active management strategies. *Physician and Sports Medicine, 24*(7), 89–93.

Condon, J. T. (1987). Psychological and physical symptoms during pregnancy: A comparison of male and female expectant parents. *Journal of Reproductive and Infant Psychology, 5,* 207–219.

Cunningham, F. G., MacDonald, P. C., & Gant, N. F. (1997). *William's obstetrics* (20th ed.). Stamford, CT: Appleton & Lange.

Davis, D. C. (1996). The discomforts of pregnancy. *Journal of Obstetric, Gynecologic, and Neonatal Nursing, 25,* 73–81.

DiIorio, C., van Lier, D., & Manteuffel, B. (1992). Patterns of nausea during the first trimester of pregnancy. *Clinical Nursing Research, 1,* 127–140.

Drake, M. L., Verhulst, D., & Fawcett, J. (1988). Physical and psychological symptoms experienced by Canadian women and their husbands during pregnancy and the postpartum. *Journal of Advanced Nursing, 13,* 436–440.

Fast, A., Weiss, L., Ducommun, E., Medina, E., & Butler, J. G. (1990). Low-back pain in pregnancy: Abdominal muscles, sit-up performance, and back pain. *Spine, 15,* 28–30.

Fawcett, J., & York, R. (1986). Spouses' physical and psychological symptoms during pregnancy and the postpartum. *Nursing Research, 35,* 144–148.

Gjerdingen, D. K., Froberg, D. G., & Kochevar, L. (1991). Changes in women's mental and physical health from pregnancy through six months postpartum. *Journal of Family Practice, 32*(2), 1–6.

Goffman, E. (1961). *Encounters.* Indianapolis, IN: Bobbs-Merrill.

Gulick, E. E., Shaw, V., & Allison, M. (1989). Dietary practices and pregnancy discomforts among urban Blacks. *Journal of Perinatology, 9,* 271–280.

Hall, S. L. (1991). *The development of self-concept during the three trimesters of pregnancy.* Unpublished doctoral dissertation, University of Texas, Austin.

Horns, P. N., Ratcliffe, L. P., Leggett, J. C., & Swanson, M. S. (1995). Pregnancy outcome among active and sedentary primiparous women. *Journal of Obstetric, Gynecologic, and Neonatal Nursing, 25,* 49–54.

Hyde, E. (1989). Acupressure therapy for morning sickness: A controlled clinical trial. *Journal of Nurse Midwifery, 34,* 171–178.

Imle, M. A. (1990). Third trimester concerns of expectant parents in transition to parenthood. *Holistic Nursing Practice, 4*(3), 25–36.

Kelley, M. A., & Boyle, J. S. (1995). How much is too much? A study of pregnant women in service industry jobs. *Journal of Obstetric, Gynecologic, and Neonatal Nursing, 24,* 269–275.

Kristiansson, P., Svardsudd, K., & von Schoultz, B. (1996). Back pain during pregnancy: A prospective study. *Spine, 21,* 702–709.

Lee, K. A., & DeJoseph, J. F. (1992). Sleep disturbances, vitality, and fatigue among a select group of employed childbearing women. *Birth, 19,* 208–213.

Lee, K. A., Hicks, G., & Nino-Murcia, G. (1991). Validity and reliability of a scale to assess fatigue. *Psychiatry Research, 36,* 291–298.

Lee, K. A., Lentz, M. J., Taylor, D. L., Mitchell, E. S., & Woods, N. F. (1994). Fatigue as a response to environmental demands in women's lives. *Image: Journal of Nursing Scholarship, 26,* 149–154.

Lee, K. A., & Zaffke, M. (1999). Longitudinal changes in fatigue and energy during pregnancy and the postpartum period. *Journal of Obstetric, Gynecologic and Neonatal Nursing, 28,* 183–191.

Lerum, C. W., & LoBiondo-Wood, G. (1989). The relationship of maternal age, quickening, and physical symptoms of pregnancy to the development of maternal-fetal attachment. *Birth: Issues in Perinatal Care and Education, 16,* 13–17.

Lips, H. M. (1985). A longitudinal study of the reporting of emotional and somatic symptoms during and after pregnancy. *Social Science and Medicine, 21,* 631–640.

McRae, M. G. (1990). *Adaptation to pregnancy and motherhood: Personality characteristics of primiparas aged 30 years and older.* Unpublished doctoral dissertation, Boston University. (*Dissertation Abstracts International, 51,* 3326B, 1991.)

Milligan, R. A., & Pugh, L. C. (1994). Fatigue during the childbearing period. In J. J. Fitzpatrick & J. S. Stevenson (Eds.), *Annual review of nursing research* (Vol. 12, pp. 33–49). New York: Springer Publishing.

Mindell, J. A., & Jacobson, B. J. (2000). Sleep disturbances during pregnancy. *Journal of Obstetric, Gynecologic, and Neonatal Nursing, 29,* 590–597.

Nuwayhid, K. A. (1984). Role function: Theory and development. In C. Roy, *Introduction to nursing: An adaptation model* (2nd ed., pp. 284–305). Englewood Cliffs, NJ: Prentice-Hall.

O'Brien, B., & Naber, S. (1992). Nausea and vomiting during pregnancy: Effects on the quality of women's lives. *Birth, 19,* 138–143.

O'Brien, B., Relyea, M. J., & Taerum, T. (1996). Efficacy of P6 acupressure in the treatment of nausea and vomiting during pregnancy. *American Journal of Obstetrics and Gynecology, 174,* 708–715.

Östgaard, H. C., Andersson, G. B. J., & Karlsson, K. (1991). Prevalence of back pain in pregnancy. *Spine, 16,* 549–552.

Östgaard, H. C., Zetherström, G., Roos-Hansson, E., & Svanberg, B. (1994). Reduction of back and posterior pelvic pain in pregnancy. *Spine, 19,* 894–900.

Parsons, T., & Shils, E. (Eds.) (1951). *Toward a general theory of action.* Cambridge: Harvard University Press.

Piers, L. S., Diggavi, S. N., Thangam, S., van Raaij, J. M. A., Shetty, P. S., & Hautvast, J. G. A. (1995). Changes in energy expenditure, anthropometry, and energy intake during the course of pregnancy and lactation in well-nourished Indian women. *American Journal of Clinical Nutrition, 61,* 501–513.

Pillitteri, A. (1998). *Maternal and child health nursing: Care of the childbearing and childrearing family* (3rd ed.). Philadelphia: Lippincott-Raven.

Pugh, L. C., & Milligan, R. (1993). A framework for the study of childbearing fatigue. *Advances in Nursing Science, 15*(4), 60–70.

Pugh, L. C., & Milligan, R. A. (1995). Patterns of fatigue during childbearing. *Applied Nursing Research, 8,* 140–146.

Reeder, S. J., Martin, L. L., & Koniak-Griffin, D. (1997). *Maternity nursing: Family, newborn, and women's health care* (18th ed.). Philadelphia: Lippincott-Raven.

Reeves, N., Potempa, K., & Gallo, A. (1991). Fatigue in early pregnancy: An exploratory study. *Journal of Nurse-Midwifery, 36,* 303–309.

Richmond, T., McCorkle, R., Tulman, L., & Fawcett, J. (1997). Measuring function. In M. Frank-Stromborg & S. J. Olsen (Eds.), *Instruments for clinical health-care research* (2nd ed., pp. 75–85). Boston: Jones and Bartlett.

Roy, C. (1984). *Introduction to nursing: An adaptation model* (2nd ed.). Englewood Cliffs, NJ: Prentice-Hall.

Schramm, W. F., Stockbauer, J. W., & Hoffman, H. J. (1996). Exercise, employment, other daily activities, and adverse pregnancy outcomes. *American Journal of Epidemiology, 143,* 211–218.

Tulman, L., Higgins, K., Fawcett, J., Nunno, C., Vansickel, C., Haas, M. B., & Speca, M. M. (1991). The Inventory of Functional Status-Antepartum Period: Development and testing. *Journal of Nurse-Midwifery, 36,* 117–123.

Turner, R. H. (1978). The role and the person. *American Journal of Sociology, 84,* 1–23.

van Lier, D., Manteuffel, B., DiIorio, C., & Stalcup, M. (1993). Nausea and fatigue during early pregnancy. *Birth, 20,* 193–197.

Wildschut, H. I. J., Harker, L. M., & Riddoch, C. J. (1993). The potential value of a short self-completion questionnaire for the assessment of habitual physical activity in pregnancy. *Journal of Psychosomatic Obstetrics and Gynecology, 14,* 17–29.

3

Weight Gain and Functioning During Pregnancy

Very low or excessive weight at the start of pregnancy, as well as very low or excessive weight gain during pregnancy, are associated with obstetrical complications during pregnancy and birth (Cogswell, Serdula, Hungerford, & Yip, 1995; Edwards, Hellerstedt, Alton, Story, & Himes, 1996) and neonatal morbidity and mortality (Naeye, 1990; Parker & Abrams, 1992; Seidman, Ever-Hadani, & Gale, 1989; Varma, 1984). Little information is available, however, on how a pregnant woman's body weight affects her adaptation during pregnancy.

In this chapter, we continue our exploration of physical health during pregnancy by focusing on the women's prepregnancy weight and weight gain during pregnancy and their relation to physical health variables and functional status within our Theory of Adaptation During Childbearing. We view prepregnancy weight and weight gain during pregnancy as focal stimuli that affect the adaptation responses of physical symptoms, physical energy, and functional status (Figures 3.1 and 3.2). Our view of body weight as a focal stimulus in this analysis is consistent with Roy's (1984) contention that one adaptation response can be viewed as a stimulus for another response. In keeping with the Roy Adaptation Model and the available evidence from the literature, we proposed that prepregnancy weight classification would be related to functional status, physical symptoms, and physical energy during each trimester of pregnancy, and that weight gained during pregnancy would be related to third trimester functional status, physical symptoms, and physical energy (Figure 3.2).

WEIGHT CLASSIFICATION AND WEIGHT GAIN DURING PREGNANCY

Body weight typically is classified using the Body Mass Index (BMI), calculated by dividing weight in kilograms by height in meters squared

This chapter is adapted from Tulman, L., Morin, K. H., & Fawcett, J. (1998). Prepregnant weight and weight gain during pregnancy: Relationship to functional status, symptoms, and energy. *Journal of Obstetric, Gynecologic, and Neonatal Nursing, 27,* 629–634.

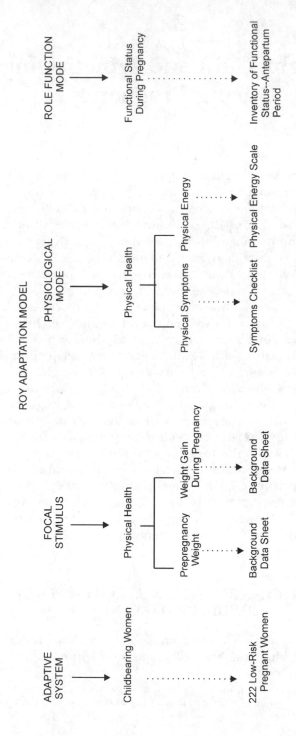

FIGURE 3.1 Linkages between the Roy Adaptation Model, physical health and functional status, and study variables and measures: Examination of the influence of prepregnancy and pregnancy body weight.

Roy Adaptation Model:

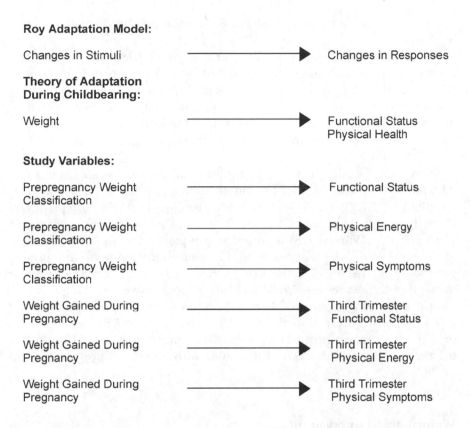

FIGURE 3.2 **Diagrams of propositions of the Roy Adaptation Model, the Theory of Adaptation During Childbearing, and pregnancy weight variables.**

(wt[Kg]/ht[m^2]) (Institute of Medicine, 1990). The standards for underweight, normal weight, and overweight for nonpregnant adults are, respectively, BMI < 19.8, BMI = 19.8–26.0, and BMI > 26.0; the standard for obesity is BMI > 29.0 (Institute of Medicine, 1990). The recommended weight gain during pregnancy for women of normal weight at the start of pregnancy is between 25 and 35 pounds. The recommended gain for underweight women is 28 to 40 pounds, and between 15 and 25 pounds for overweight women (Institute of Medicine, 1990; Keppel & Taffel, 1993; Wolfe & Gross, 1994).

Many researchers have studied weight gain during pregnancy. For example, Brewer, Bates, and Vannoy (1989) reported an average weight gain of 33 pounds in a group of 56 women. Dewey, Heinig, and Nommsen (1993) reported that a group of 85 women gained an average of 35 pounds.

Ranjitkar's (1991) data revealed that a group of 108 women gained an average of 32 pounds, with a range of 10 to 75 pounds. Using the BMI to classify weight, Ranjitkar reported that among a group of 301 women surveyed after childbirth, the 68 underweight women gained an average of 32.78 pounds, the 166 normal weight women gained an average of 33.88 pounds, and the 5 overweight women gained an average of 18.04 pounds.

Dawes and Grudzinskas (1991) reported an average weight gain of 23.6 pounds in a sample of 1,145 women; initially heavy (> 149.6 pounds) and light (< 121.9 pounds) women gained less weight during pregnancy than their initially medium weight (132–149.6 pounds) counterparts. More recently, Wiles (1998) reported weight gains of up to 72.6 pounds at 30 weeks of pregnancy among 37 overweight women; the pre-pregnancy BMI scores for the women ranged from 25 to 45, with an average of 32. Moreover, Walker (1998) reported average pregnancy weight gains ranging from 28.38 to 39.82 pounds among a group of 227 women who were classified according to their level of satisfaction or distress with their postpartum weight. The prepregnancy BMI scores for the women ranged from 21.6 to 26.6, with an overall average BMI of 23.5.

Weight and Functional Status

Weight has been linked to functional status in nonpregnant popula-tions. Stewart and Brook (1983) assessed functional status in a healthy sample of 2,438 men and 2,749 women. They found that 19% of normal weight persons, 28% of moderately overweight persons, and 34% of severely overweight persons experienced limitations in personal func-tioning, defined as mobility and performance of self-care activities. Furthermore, 13% of moderately overweight persons and 16% of se-verely overweight persons experienced limitations in role functioning, defined as performance of occupational or educational activities, whereas the incidence of limited role functioning for persons weighing within the recommended range was 12%. Platte and colleagues (1995) found that nonpregnant individuals who were excessively overweight used more energy to perform physical activities than normal weight individuals. Coakley and colleagues (1998) reported that increasing levels of Body Mass Index were associated with reduced physical function in a sample of 56,510 women 45 to 71 years of age.

No specific literature addressing the effects of initial weight or pregnancy weight gain on functional status during pregnancy was available. We sought to extend knowledge by examining the relation of prepregnancy weight classification to functional status during each trimester, as well as the relation of weight gained during pregnancy to third trimester functional status.

Weight and Physical Symptoms

As noted in chapter 2, a considerable amount of research already has focused on the incidence of physical discomforts or symptoms during pregnancy. Surprisingly, we were unable to locate any studies that addressed the relation of a pregnant woman's body weight to physical symptoms, including the frequently occurring symptoms of back pain, nausea, and vomiting. This part of our study, therefore, included an analysis of the relation of prepregnancy weight classification to the number and type of physical symptoms experienced during each trimester, as well as the relation of weight gained during pregnancy to third trimester physical symptoms.

Weight and Physical Energy

Fatigue and stamina during pregnancy have been studied, and preliminary hypotheses have been developed about their association with weight gain. Poole (1986) theorized that fatigue results from depleted energy stores that typically occur during pregnancy. Pugh and Milligan (1993) speculated that several physiological, psychological, and situational factors predispose to fatigue. Although not operationally defined, and not supported empirically, excessive weight gain was considered a contributing physiological factor. Reeves, Potempa, and Gallo (1991), however, in studying 30 low-risk women at the beginning of pregnancy, found that as weight increased, the women's stamina, defined as the inclination to embrace and value physical activity, also increased. They also found that as the women's weight increased, their fatigue decreased. In this part of our study, we focused on the relation of prepregnancy weight classification to physical energy during each trimester, and the

relation of weight gained during pregnancy to third trimester physical energy.

THE RESULTS OF OUR STUDY

Of the 227 women in our study for whom complete pregnancy data
were available, two had multiple gestations, two did not know their
weight at the first trimester interview, and one woman did not know
her weight at the third trimester interview. These five women were
excluded, yielding a sample of 222 women for the analyses presented
in this chapter.

Prepregnancy Weight Classification, Functional Status, Physical Symptoms, and Physical Energy During Pregnancy

Prepregnancy weight, as measured by BMI, ranged from 16.68 to 34.62.
Thirty-six (16%) of the women were classified as beginning the preg-
nancy as underweight (BMI < 19.8), 151 (68%) were of normal weight
(BMI 19.8–26.0), and 35 (16%) were overweight (BMI > 26.0).

There were no differences in functional status, number of physical
symptoms, or level of physical energy level among the initially underweight, normal weight, and overweight groups of women in any of the
three trimesters ($p > .05$) (Table 3.1). There also were no differences
among the three groups of women in the incidence of any specific
physical symptom ($p > .05$).

Changes in Weight During Pregnancy

We calculated weight gain during pregnancy in two ways: the difference
in pounds between prepregnancy weight and weight at the end of
a particular trimester, and the percentage of weight gained during
pregnancy (weight gain in pounds divided by prepregnancy weight).
The number of pounds gained did not differ among the initially underweight, normal weight, and overweight groups of women for any of the
three trimesters ($p > .05$). Overall, the women gained from 1 to 64
pounds during the pregnancy, with an average gain for the three trimesters of 30.65 pounds.

TABLE 3.1 Functional Status, Physical Symptoms, and Physical Energy by Prepregnancy Weight Group (*N* = 222)

	Prepregnancy Weight Group*		
	Underweight (*n* = 36)	Normal Weight (*n* = 151)	Overweight (*n* = 35)
First Trimester			
Functional Status (*M, SD*)**	2.60 (.38)	2.54 (.38)	2.54 (.32)
Number of Physical Symptoms (*M, SD*)***	8.64 (2.47)	9.00 (2.76)	8.26 (2.52)
Maintain Usual Level of Physical Energy (%)			
Not at All	14%	26%	40%
Partially	69%	61%	54%
Fully	17%	13%	6%
Second Trimester			
Functional Status (*M, SD*)**	2.68 (.28)	2.63 (.26)	2.60 (.26)
Number of Physical Symptoms (*M, SD*)***	7.83 (2.63)	9.08 (3.16)	8.54 (3.17)
Maintain Usual Level of Physical Energy (%)			
Not at All	8%	7%	14%
Partially	47%	62%	46%
Fully	45%	31%	40%
Third Trimester			
Functional Status (*M, SD*)**	2.45 (.43)	2.39 (.36)	2.34 (.37)
Number of Physical Symptoms (*M, SD*)***	9.50 (2.74)	9.72 (2.97)	9.63 (2.67)
Maintain Usual Level of Physical Energy (%)			
Not at All	28%	24%	29%
Partially	55%	63%	51%
Fully	17%	13%	20%

*No statistically significant differences among the three weight groups, *p* > .05.
**Potential range of scores = 1–3; higher scores indicate greater functional status.
***Potential range of scores = 0–21 symptoms.

In contrast, the initially underweight, normal weight, and overweight groups differed in percentage of weight gained ($p < .00005$). The initially overweight group of women gained relatively less (in percentage terms) ($M = 17\%$) than either the normal weight ($M = 24\%$) or the underweight ($M = 26\%$) groups. The three weight groups also differed on the percentage of women who gained more than the recommended amount during pregnancy ($p < .0005$). Fewer initially underweight women (6%) gained more than the upper limits of the recommended amount for their group (40 pounds) compared with 25% of normal weight women (upper limit of 35 pounds) and 57% of the overweight women (upper limit of 25 pounds).

Pregnancy Weight Gain and Functional Status

We found a difference in functional status between the women whose total weight gain for the pregnancy was more than the recommended amount based on their prepregnancy BMI ($n = 62$) and those who gained within the recommended range ($n = 160$) ($p = .014$). The women who gained an excessive amount of weight had a lower third trimester level of functional status ($M = 2.30$) than those who did not ($M = 2.43$).

When the women were interviewed six months after delivery about what could have helped them during pregnancy, more than one quarter (27%) told us that their weight had hindered performance of their usual activities at some point in the pregnancy. One woman simply stated that she "just felt that extra weight," and another stated that "carrying the weight was most uncomfortable." Another woman noted that "carrying more weight" made it difficult to be as active as she tried to be. One other woman noted that her weight gain made it "harder to stay active."

Still other women commented specifically about the impact of their large size at the end of the pregnancy on performance of their usual activities. Three women spoke for the others when they said:

> Well, it certainly got to a point in the last two and a half months that I didn't continue [my usual activities], because I was very tired and large and uncomfortable.

> Towards the end, the bulkiness of my body made it hard to do certain things.

> I continued my activities except for at the end, when I was pretty large. It was difficult then.

Pregnancy Weight Gain, Physical Symptoms, and Physical Energy

There were no differences in number of physical symptoms or level of physical energy for those women who gained an excessive amount of weight and those who did not ($p > .05$). Some women's comments, however, reflected a link between their weight and tiredness, which could be considered a proxy for physical energy. In this regard, the women noted that their performance of usual activities was hindered by:

Being tired, huge, and exhausted.

Being tired. Getting heavier.

Feeling tired and being big.

Two women were even more explicit about the link between their weight and physical energy. They stated:

The bigger the belly, the harder [it was to do anything]; my activity level slowed down. I wasn't really a high energy person [who] ran around like crazy but I started to slow down and get tired; [a] tired all day thing.

I gained a lot of weight with this baby and I felt tired, so moving became an effort.

CONCLUSION

The results for this part of our study lend some support to the credibility of the Roy Adaptation Model proposition asserting that focal stimuli influence adaptation responses and that part of our Theory of Adaptation During Childbearing addressing the influence of physical health, in the form of body weight variables, on other physical health variables (physical symptoms and physical energy) and functional status. Our finding that the focal stimulus of weight gain during pregnancy influenced functional status supports the credibility of the Roy Adaptation Model. In contrast, our findings that the focal stimulus of prepregnancy weight classification had no influence on adaptation in the physiological and role function modes during pregnancy, and that the focal stimulus of weight gain during pregnancy had no influence on adaptation in the physiological mode raise questions about the credibility of the Roy Adaptation Model.

Overall, our findings indicate that the part of our Theory of Adaptation During Childbearing addressing the influence of pregnancy weight variables should be more parsimonious. More specifically, the only empirically supported proposition asserts that pregnancy weight gain is associated with functional status (Figure 3.2). The proposition linking prepregnancy weight classification with functional status, physical symptoms, and physical energy (Figure 3.2) was not supported. Similarly, the proposition linking pregnancy weight gain with physical symptoms and physical energy (Figure 3.2) was not supported.

The average (30.65 pounds) and range (1–64 pounds) for weight gained by the women in our study is similar to the pregnancy weight gains reported by some other researchers (Ranjitkar, 1991; Walker, 1998) but higher than the average gain reported by Dawes and Grudzinskas (1991). In our study, a greater percentage of initially overweight women were more likely to gain more than the recommended amount of weight based on their prepregnancy weight classification than normal weight or underweight women. However, the *average* weight gain during pregnancy for this overweight group was similar to the *average* weight gain for the underweight and normal weight groups. This finding conflicts with other researchers' results indicating that underweight and overweight women tend to gain less weight than women who begin pregnancy at normal weight (Dawes & Grudzinskas, 1991), and that overweight women tend to gain less weight than women who begin pregnancy either underweight or at normal weight (Ekblad & Grenman, 1992; Siega-Riz, Adair, & Hobel, 1994). The similarity in weight gain among the groups in our study may be the reason why no differences were found in functional status, physical symptoms, or physical energy among the three groups. The lack of differences also may be related to the limited number of women in our study who were extremely overweight. Inasmuch as only 8% of our sample could be classified as obese (BMI > 29.0), this subcategory within the overweight group did not have a sufficient number of women to form a separate group for comparison with the other three (underweight, normal weight, overweight) groups. A sample that includes a greater number of obese women would have allowed for more detailed analysis of the effect of the focal stimulus of weight on the physiological and role function mode adaptation responses during pregnancy.

The lower level of functional status in the third trimester found among those women who gained an excessive amount of weight based on their prepregnancy weight, compared with the women with a normal weight gain, may be explained by two possible sequences of events. First, increased weight may contribute to an increase in energy expenditure for activities that, in turn, contributes to a decrease in performance of activities as an energy conservation measure. Alternatively, a decrease in performance of activities may contribute to a decrease in energy expenditure that, in turn, leads to an increase in weight. Future research should determine the order of events by evaluating weight gain, energy expenditure, and functional status each week throughout pregnancy.

The lack of a relation between weight and physical energy does not support Poole's (1986) and Pugh and Milligan's (1993) frameworks. However, physical energy as defined in our study may not be the polar opposite of fatigue as defined by Poole and Pugh and Mulligan. Further clarification of the definition and measurement of the related concepts of physical energy and fatigue is needed.

REFERENCES

Brewer, M. M., Bates, M. R., & Vannoy, L. P. (1989). Postpartum changes in maternal weight and body fat deposits in lactating versus non-lactating women. *American Journal of Clinical Nutrition, 49*, 259–265.

Coakley, E. H., Kawachi, I., Manson, J. E., Speizer, F. E., Willet, W. C., & Colditz, G. A. (1998). Lower levels of physical functioning are associated with higher body weight among middle-aged and older women. *International Journal of Obesity, 22*, 958–965.

Cogswell, M. E., Serdula, M. K., Hungerford, D. W., & Yip, R. (1995). Gestational weight gain among average-weight and overweight women: What is excessive? *American Journal of Obstetrics and Gynecology, 172*, 705–712.

Dawes, M. G., & Grudzinskas, J. G. (1991). Patterns of maternal weight gain in pregnancy. *British Journal of Obstetrics and Gynaecology, 98*, 195–201.

Dewey, K. G., Heinig, M. J., & Nommsen, L. A. (1993). Maternal weight-loss patterns during prolonged lactation. *American Journal of Clinical Nutrition, 58*, 162–166.

Edwards, L. E., Hellerstedt, W. L., Alton, I. R., Story, M., & Himes, J. H. (1996). Pregnancy complications and birth outcomes in obese and normal-weight women: Effects of gestational weight change. *Obstetrics and Gynecology, 87*, 389–394.

Ekblad, U., & Grenman, S. (1992). Maternal weight, weight gain during pregnancy and pregnancy outcome. *International Journal of Gynecology and Obstetrics, 39*, 277–283.

Institute of Medicine. (1990). *Nutrition during pregnancy: Weight gain and nutrients.* Washington, DC: National Academy Press.

Keppel, K. G., & Taffel, S. M. (1993). Pregnancy-related weight gain and retention: Implications of the 1990 Institute of Medicine guidelines. *American Journal of Public Health, 83*, 1100–1103.

Naeye, R. L. (1990). Maternal body weight and pregnancy outcome. *American Journal of Clinical Nutrition, 52,* 273–279.

Parker, J. D., & Abrams, B. (1992). Prenatal weight gain advice: An examination of the recent prenatal weight gain recommendations of the Institute of Medicine. *Obstetrics and Gynecology, 79,* 664–669.

Platte, P., Pirke, F. M., Wade, S. E., Trimborn, P., & Fichter, M. N. (1995). Physical activity, total energy expenditure, and food intake in grossly obese and normal weight women. *International Journal of Eating Disorders, 17,* 51–57.

Poole, C. J. (1986). Fatigue during the first trimester of pregnancy. *Journal of Obstetric, Gynecologic, and Neonatal Nurses, 15,* 375–379.

Pugh, L. C., & Milligan, R. A. (1993). A framework for the study of childbearing fatigue. *Advances in Nursing Science, 15*(4), 60–70.

Ranjitkar, M. L. (1991). *Weight gain recommendations in pregnancy and their effects on pregnancy outcomes.* Unpublished doctoral thesis, Tufts University.

Reeves, N., Potempa, K., & Gallo, A. (1991). Fatigue in early pregnancy. *Journal of Nurse-Midwifery, 36,* 303–309.

Roy, C. (1984). *Introduction to nursing: An adaptation model* (2nd ed.). Englewood Cliffs, NJ: Prentice-Hall.

Seidman, D. S., Ever-Hadani, P., & Gale, R. (1989). The effect of maternal weight gain in pregnancy on birth weight. *Obstetrics & Gynecology, 74,* 240–246.

Siega-Riz, A. M., Adair, L. S., & Hobel, C. J. (1994). Institute of Medicine maternal weight gain recommendations and pregnancy outcome in a predominately Hispanic population. *Obstetrics and Gynecology, 84,* 565–573.

Stewart, A. J., & Brook, R. H. (1983). Effects of being overweight. *American Journal of Public Health, 73,* 171–178.

Varma, T. R. (1984). Maternal weight and weight gain in pregnancy and obstetric outcome. *International Journal of Gynaecology and Obstetrics, 22,* 161–166.

Walker, L. O. (1998). Weight-related distress in the early months after childbirth. *Western Journal of Nursing Research, 20,* 30–44.

Wiles, R. (1998). The views of women of above average weight about appropriate weight gain in pregnancy. *Midwifery, 14,* 254–260.

Wolfe, H. M., & Gross, T. L. (1994). Obesity in pregnancy. *Clinics in Obstetrics and Gynecology, 37,* 596–604.

4

Anticipating Delivery and Motherhood

As we pointed out in chapter 2, little is known about the subtle changes experienced by low-risk pregnant women as they adapt during childbearing. In this chapter, we present the part of our Theory of Adaptation During Childbearing dealing with psychosocial health, family relationships, and functional status during pregnancy (Figures 4.1 and 4.2). Here, we continue to examine adaptation, as experienced by low-risk pregnant women during the three trimesters of pregnancy, by focusing on their psychosocial health and family relationships. In keeping with the Roy Adaptation Model and the available evidence from the literature, we proposed that several psychosocial health variables would change during pregnancy, including psychological symptoms (feeling anxious, feeling depressed, feeling better than usual); acceptance of pregnancy; identification of a motherhood role; preparation for labor; fear of pain, helplessness, and loss of control during labor; and concern for well-being of self and baby (Figure 4.2 [A]). We also proposed that two family relationships variables—relationship with mother and relationship with husband—would change during pregnancy (Figure 4.2 [A]). Furthermore, we proposed that all of those psychosocial health variables and family relationships variables would be related to functional status during each trimester of pregnancy (Figure 4.2 [B, C]).

PSYCHOSOCIAL HEALTH DURING PREGNANCY

Pregnancy is certainly a physical experience but, according to Schroeder-Zwelling (1988), "is most often defined as a psychological or emotional experience" (p. 39). Accordingly, our study included variables that reflect psychosocial health during pregnancy.

Psychological Symptoms

Newton (1955), as part of a now classic study of 123 postpartum women, examined feelings about pregnancy. She found that women had both

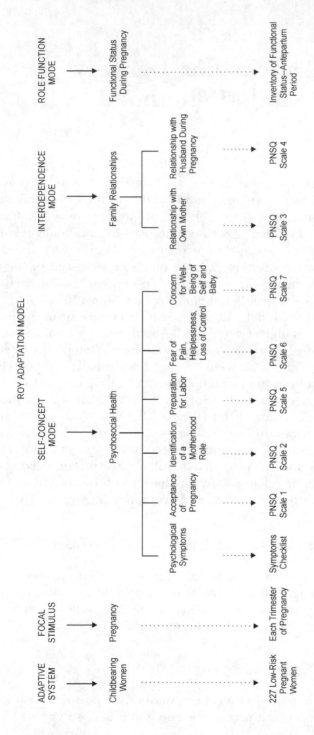

FIGURE 4.1 Linkages between the Roy Adaptation Model, psychosocial health, family relationships, and functional status, and study variables and measures.

Legend: PNSQ = Prenatal Self-Evaluation Questionnaire

ROY ADAPTATION MODEL

ADAPTIVE SYSTEM

FOCAL STIMULUS

SELF-CONCEPT MODE

INTERDEPENDENCE MODE

ROLE FUNCTION MODE

Childbearing Women

Pregnancy

Psychosocial Health

Family Relationships

Functional Status During Pregnancy

Psychological Symptoms

Acceptance of Pregnancy

Identification of a Motherhood Role

Preparation for Labor

Fear of Pain, Helplessness, Loss of Control

Concern for Well-Being of Self and Baby

Relationship with Own Mother

Relationship with Husband During Pregnancy

Symptoms Checklist

PNSQ Scale 1

PNSQ Scale 2

PNSQ Scale 5

PNSQ Scale 6

PNSQ Scale 7

PNSQ Scale 3

PNSQ Scale 4

Inventory of Functional Status—Antepartum Period

227 Low-Risk Pregnant Women

Each Trimester of Pregnancy

44

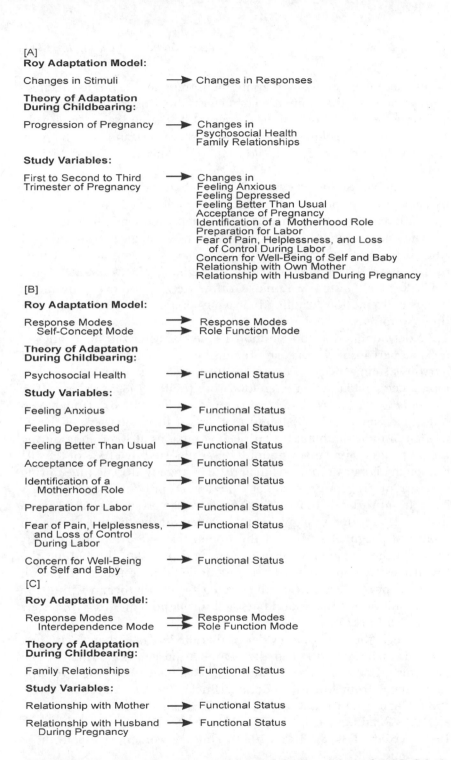

[A]
Roy Adaptation Model:

Changes in Stimuli ———▶ Changes in Responses

**Theory of Adaptation
During Childbearing:**

Progression of Pregnancy ———▶ Changes in
Psychosocial Health
Family Relationships

Study Variables:

First to Second to Third ———▶ Changes in
Trimester of Pregnancy   Feeling Anxious
Feeling Depressed
Feeling Better Than Usual
Acceptance of Pregnancy
Identification of a Motherhood Role
Preparation for Labor
Fear of Pain, Helplessness, and Loss
of Control During Labor
Concern for Well-Being of Self and Baby
Relationship with Own Mother
Relationship with Husband During Pregnancy

[B]
Roy Adaptation Model:

Response Modes ———▶ Response Modes
Self-Concept Mode ———▶ Role Function Mode

**Theory of Adaptation
During Childbearing:**

Psychosocial Health ———▶ Functional Status

Study Variables:

Feeling Anxious ———▶ Functional Status

Feeling Depressed ———▶ Functional Status

Feeling Better Than Usual ———▶ Functional Status

Acceptance of Pregnancy ———▶ Functional Status

Identification of a ———▶ Functional Status
Motherhood Role

Preparation for Labor ———▶ Functional Status

Fear of Pain, Helplessness, ———▶ Functional Status
and Loss of Control
During Labor

Concern for Well-Being ———▶ Functional Status
of Self and Baby

[C]

Roy Adaptation Model:

Response Modes ———▶ Response Modes
Interdependence Mode ———▶ Role Function Mode

**Theory of Adaptation
During Childbearing:**

Family Relationships ———▶ Functional Status

Study Variables:

Relationship with Mother ———▶ Functional Status

Relationship with Husband ———▶ Functional Status
During Pregnancy

**FIGURE 4.2 Diagrams of propositions of the Roy Adaptation Model, the
Theory of Adaptation During Childbearing, and study variables: Functional
status, psychosocial health, and family relationships during pregnancy.**

positive and negative feelings about their pregnancies. Positive feelings were evident in the women's characterizations of their pregnancies as "pretty good," "no trouble," "wonderful," "swell," and "real well" (p. 27). Negative feelings were evident in characterizations of the pregnancy as "not too good," "all right but . . . ," "miserable," and "sick all the time" (p. 27).

Our study extended beyond feelings about pregnancy to specific psychological symptoms associated with childbearing. We were especially interested the symptoms of anxiety, depression, and feeling better than usual. We selected those particular psychological symptoms for study based on their description in textbooks as "common complaints" or symptoms during pregnancy (Cunningham, MacDonald, & Gant, 1997; Reeder, Martin, & Koniak-Griffin, 1997). Moreover, the mood swings and emotional lability that typify pregnancy encompass those three symptoms.

Anxiety, defined as "an emotional state characterized by feelings of tension, nervousness, worry, apprehension, and heightened autonomic nervous system activity" (Lederman, 1984, p. 28), is regarded as a common aspect of adaptation to childbearing (Leifer, 1980; Newton, 1955; Uddenberg, Fagerström, & Hakanson-Zaunders, 1976). Drake, Verhulst, and Fawcett (1988) found that almost three quarters of the 20 women in their sample reported feeling anxious at some time during the pregnancy. Similarly, Condon (1987) reported that 61% of the 101 women in his study reported an increase in anxiety at some time during the current pregnancy over that experienced prior to the pregnancy. Fawcett and York (1986) found that anxiety was a psychological symptom frequently reported by a group of 23 women during the third to fourth month of pregnancy. Most of the women indicated that the anxiety began in the first month of pregnancy and persisted throughout the first trimester. A group of 24 women queried during the ninth month of pregnancy indicated that the feeling of anxiety began within the first month of pregnancy and persisted throughout all three trimesters (Fawcett & York, 1986).

Although there is some evidence that anxiety is higher in the first and third trimesters than in the second trimester (Lederman, 1984; Lederman, Harrison, & Worsham, 1993; Reading, 1983), the level typically ranges from low to moderate (Buckwalter et al., 1999; Glazer, 1980; Hughes, Turton, & Evans, 1999; Lederman, 1984; Lederman et al., 1993; Reading, 1983; Rini, Dunkel-Schetter, Wadhwa, & Sandman, 1999; Teixeira, Fisk, & Glover, 1999). Thus few women, especially those experiencing low-risk pregnancies, report a high level of anxiety at any time during pregnancy. More specifically, Teixeira and colleagues (1999) reported that just 15 of the 100 third trimester women in their study experienced a high level of anxiety. Moreover, although Condon (1987) found that women reported an increase in anxiety during pregnancy relative to the nonpregnant state, Behrenz and Monga (1999) found that the relatively low level of anxiety experienced by first trimester pregnant women did not differ from that experienced by their nonpregnant counterparts.

Depression, generally regarded as a negative feeling state involving diminished interest or pleasure in usual activities, along with "thoughts of giving up or hopelessness about the future" (Affonso, Liu-Chiang, & Mayberry, 1999, p. 230), also is a frequently reported symptom during pregnancy (Condon, 1987; Drake, Verhulst, & Fawcett, 1988; Fawcett & York, 1986; Gotlib, Wiffen, Mount, Milne, & Cordy, 1989; Zajicek & Wolkind, 1978). Kaplan (1986) argued that "depression may be viewed as one of several normal affective developments of pregnancy rooted in some of the physiological events of gestation" (p. 35). Affonso, Lovett, Paul, and Sheptak (1990) pointed out that the physical symptoms of pregnancy typically mimic the symptoms of depression, leading to both overdiagnosis and underdiagnosis of clinical depression during pregnancy.

Pregnant women have reported that their feelings of depression began in the first month of pregnancy and persisted throughout all three trimesters (Fawcett & York, 1986; Affonso et al., 1993). Evidence regarding changes in depression vary. Some investigators have reported no appreciable changes during the three trimesters of pregnancy (Lederman, 1984), whereas others have found evidence of a slight decrease in depression from the first to the third trimester (Lederman, Harrison, & Worsham, 1993). Low-risk pregnant women typically experience mild to moderate levels of depression (Affonso et al., 1992; Buckwalter et al., 1999; Fawcett & York, 1986; Gjerdingen, Froberg, & Kochevar, 1991; Hughes, Turton, & Evans, 1999; Lederman, Harrison, & Worsham, 1993; Lederman, Harrison, & Worsham, 1994; Lips, 1985) that do not differ from levels experienced by nonpregnant women (Behrenz & Monga, 1999; Grush & Cohen, 1998; Kaplan, 1986). Indeed, researchers have reported a high level of depression in just 5% to 10% of low-risk pregnant women (Affonso et al., 1992; Gotlib, Wiffen, Mount, Milne, & Cordy, 1989; Hughes, Turton, & Evans, 1999; O'Hara, 1986). Those woman should more appropriately be classified as having a high-risk pregnancy (Haglund & Britton, 1998).

Feeling better than usual is another psychological symptom reported by some women during pregnancy (Drake, Verhulst, & Fawcett, 1988; Fawcett & York, 1987). This symptom is similar to a sense of well-being, which has been defined as the individual's perception of life satisfaction and health (White, 1992). Although we did not locate any longitudinal studies of changes in feeling better than usual during pregnancy, we speculated that this psychological symptom would be experienced more frequently during the second trimester than the first or third trimesters. We based our speculation on the observation that the second trimester is a "quiescent period of least physiological and psychological stresses associated with childbearing" (Arizmendi & Affonso, 1987, p. 747). In addition, Reeder and colleagues (1997) noted that the feeling of well-being is characteristic of the second trimester. They attributed that feeling to a decrease in the physical symptoms, fear, and anxiety that are typical during the first trimester.

PNSQ Psychosocial Health Variables

Our interest in psychosocial health during pregnancy extended to several other variables, including the woman's acceptance of her pregnancy; her identification of a motherhood role; her feelings regarding preparation for labor; her fear of pain, helplessness, and loss of control during labor; and her concern for the well-being of herself and her baby. All of these variables are measured by the *Prenatal Self-Evaluation Questionnaire* (PNSQ); the definition of each variable is given in the Appendix (Table A.1). Our review of studies using the PNSQ and other instruments that measure similar variables revealed that pregnant women typically report relatively positive evaluations of those aspects of psychosocial health (Arizmendi & Affonso, 1987; Gottesman, 1992; Hall, 1991; Halman, Oakley, & Lederman, 1995; Lederman, 1996; Lederman, Harrison, & Worsham, 1993, 1994; Lederman & Lederman, 1996; Lederman & Miller, 1998; Randell, 1988; Rini, Dunkel-Schetter, Wadhwa, & Sandman, 1999; Stark, 1997).

Most of these studies focused on women during just the third trimester of pregnancy. Randell (1988), however, administered the PNSQ to 14 primiparous women during the first and third trimesters. Examination of the mean scores revealed that acceptance of pregnancy and identification of a motherhood role increased from the first to the third trimester. Hall (1991) administered the PNSQ to 32 primiparas during each trimester of pregnancy. She found statistical evidence of changes across the three trimesters in acceptance of pregnancy, identification of a motherhood role, feelings regarding preparation for labor, and fear of pain, helplessness, and loss of control during labor. Further analysis of the data revealed that the women's acceptance of the pregnancy increased significantly from the second to the third trimester, as did their feelings regarding preparation for labor. Moreover, fear of pain, helplessness, and loss of control during labor decreased from the first to the second trimester (Hall, 1991). Lederman, Harrison, and Worsham (1993, 1994) administered the PNSQ to almost 700 women during each trimester of pregnancy. They found statistical evidence of an increase in the women's acceptance of pregnancy and in feelings regarding preparation for labor from the first to the third trimester. They also found statistical evidence of a decrease in fear of pain, helplessness, and loss of control during labor from the second to the third trimester. The women's concern for the well-being of herself and her baby was highest during the second trimester and lowest in the third trimester (Lederman, Harrison, & Worsham, 1993).

Psychosocial Health and Functional Status

A large number of studies have focused on the relation between psychosocial health and complications during pregnancy, progress in labor, infant birth weight, and postpartum adaptation (Lederman, 1984, 1986; Lederman, Harrison, & Worsham, 1993; Reading, 1983). We located just one study that focused on the relation between depression and such health behaviors as diet/eating, substance abuse, recklessness, hygiene practices, sleep/rest, and exercise (Walker, Cooney, & Riggs, 1999); findings indicated that higher levels of depressive symptoms were associated with less favorable health behaviors in early pregnancy. The influence of several psychosocial health variables on functional status during pregnancy, however, had not been explored prior to our study.

FAMILY RELATIONSHIPS DURING PREGNANCY

Our interest in family relationships during pregnancy centered on the woman's relationship with her own mother and her relationship with her husband. Both variables are measured by the PNSQ; the definitions are given in the Appendix (Table A.1). Our review of relevant studies revealed that low-risk pregnant women typically report relatively positive evaluations of their relationships with their mothers and husbands, at least by the third trimester (Arizmendi & Affonso, 1987; Gottesman, 1992; Hall, 1991; Halman, Oakley, & Lederman, 1995; Lederman & Lederman, 1996; Lederman & Miller, 1998; Randell, 1988; Stark, 1997; Zachariah, 1994a, 1994b).

Inspection of the mean scores in Randell's (1988) study of 14 primiparas revealed that a woman's relationship with her own mother and her relationship with her husband improved from the first to the third trimester. In contrast, Hall (1991) and Lederman, Harrison, and Worsham (1993) reported no statistical evidence of changes in women's relationships with their own mothers or their husbands from the first to the second or the third trimester of pregnancy. Using qualitative methodology, Richardson (1981) found that pregnant women's relationships with their parents and their husbands changed from early to midpregnancy and then became stable during the latter half of pregnancy.

Family Relationships and Functional Status

The influence of family relationships on functional status during pregnancy has not yet been fully explored. The woman's relationship with her mother is thought to be an important factor in her identification with the maternal role; the correlations between relationship with mother and pregnancy adaptation have, however, ranged from low to moderate in magnitude (Lederman & Lederman, 1996). Furthermore, although clinicians typically regard the woman's relationship with her husband as an important area of assessment (Haglund & Britton, 1998), the influence of the marital relationship on adaptation to pregnancy is unclear. Studies guided by crisis theory have linked the quality of the marital relationship with transition to parenthood (Hobbs, 1965; Hobbs & Cole, 1976). However, an integrative research review revealed conflicting findings for correlations between measures of the quality of the marital relationship and pregnancy adaptation (Lederman & Lederman, 1996).

THE RESULTS OF OUR STUDY

We examined the data from the 227 women in our study for changes in psychosocial health and family relationships during pregnancy (Table

4.1). We also looked at the correlations of variables reflecting psychological symptoms, psychosocial health and family relationships with functional status for each trimester (Table 4.2). [See our data for functional status in chapter 2 (Table 2.1).] In addition, we examined the women's responses to interviews we conducted six months after delivery. They told us how their psychosocial health and their family relationships either helped them to continue or hindered them from continuing their usual activities during pregnancy.

Changes in Psychological Symptoms

The data for each psychological symptom—feeling anxious, feeling depressed, and feeling better than usual—revealed some changes during the three trimesters of pregnancy (Table 4.1). One half (50%) of the women reported feeling anxious in the first trimester; slightly more than two fifths (42%) reported this symptom in the second trimester; and more than one half (55%), in the third trimester. No statistical evidence of a change in this symptom was evident from the first to the second trimester. A statistically significant change was, however, evident from the second to the third trimester ($p = .002$).

Slightly more than one fifth of the women reported feeling depressed each trimester—25% in the first trimester, 22% in the second, and 20% in the third (Table 4.1). There were no statistically significant changes in this symptom throughout the three trimesters of pregnancy.

As can be seen in Table 4.1, slightly more than one eighth (13%) of the women reported feeling better than usual during the first trimester. The percentage doubled to more than one quarter (26%) in the second trimester, and then decreased to less than one fifth (19%) in the third trimester. The only statistically significant change in this symptom, however, was from the first to the second trimester ($p < .0005$).

Psychological Symptoms and Functional Status

The correlations between the three psychological symptoms and functional status were of relatively low magnitude (Table 4.2). The negative correlation between feeling anxious and functional status was statistically significant during each trimester ($p < .05$); women who reported feeling anxious performed their usual activities at a lower level throughout pregnancy than did their counterparts who did not report feeling

TABLE 4.1   Changes in Psychosocial Health Variables and Family Relationship Variables During Pregnancy (*N* = 227)

Variable	First Trimester	Second Trimester	Third Trimester	*p*
Psychological Symptoms [%]				
FEELING ANXIOUS	50%	42%	55%	.005[b]
FEELING DEPRESSED	25%	22%	20%	.436
FEELING BETTER THAN USUAL	13%	26%	19%	< .0005[a]
Prenatal Self-Evaluation Questionnaire Psychosocial Health Variables [*M, SD*]				
ACCEPTANCE OF PREGNANCY*	22.81 (7.07)	21.12 (6.75)	21.69 (6.59)	< .0005[a]
IDENTIFICATION OF A MOTHERHOOD ROLE**	21.74 (4.80)	21.62 (4.72)	21.23 (4.7)	.04[d]
PREPARATION FOR LABOR***	17.58 (5.23)	17.22 (4.91)	15.76 (4.37)	< .0005[b]
FEAR OF PAIN, HELPLESSNESS, AND LOSS OF CONTROL DURING LABOR***	16.81 (3.92)	17.05 (3.90)	16.68 (4.01)	.071
CONCERN FOR WELL-BEING OF SELF AND BABY***	16.13 (4.67)	16.18 (4.23)	16.09 (4.59)	.890
Prenatal Self-Evaluation Questionnaire Family Relationship Variables [*M, SD*]				
RELATIONSHIP WITH MOTHER***	18.02 (6.56)	18.18 (6.58)	18.21 (6.86)	.885
RELATIONSHIP WITH HUSBAND***	14.69 (3.85)	16.22 (4.21)	15.89 (4.06)	< .0005[a]

[a]Difference between first trimester and second trimester statistically significant.
[b]Difference between second trimester and third trimester statistically significant.
[c]Differences between first trimester and second trimester and second trimester and third trimester statistically significant.
[d]Differences between trimesters not statistically significant.
*Potential range of scores = 14–56; lower scores indicate more positive evaluation.
**Potential range of scores = 15–60; lower scores indicate more positive evaluation.
***Potential range of scores = 10–40; lower scores indicate more positive evaluation.

TABLE 4.2 **Correlations of Psychosocial Health and Family Relationship Variables With Functional Status During Pregnancy** (*N* = 227)

Variable	First Trimester Functional Status	Second Trimester Functional Status	Third Trimester Functional Status
Psychological Symptoms			
FEELING ANXIOUS	−.169*	−.239***	−.286***
FEELING DEPRESSED	−.251***	−.133*	−.286***
FEELING BETTER THAN USUAL	.191**	−.004	.075
Prenatal Self-Evaluation Questionnaire Psychosocial Health Variables			
ACCEPTANCE OF PREGNANCY	−.295***	−.309***	−.205***
IDENTIFICATION OF A MOTHERHOOD ROLE	−.089	−.147*	−.016
PREPARATION FOR LABOR	−.300***	−.121	−.161*
FEAR OF PAIN, HELPLESSNESS, AND LOSS OF CONTROL DURING LABOR	−.265***	−.277***	−.213**
CONCERN FOR WELL-BEING OF SELF AND BABY	−.182**	−.214**	−.201**
Prenatal Self-Evaluation Questionnaire Family Relationship Variables			
RELATIONSHIP WITH MOTHER	−.005	−.053	.049
RELATIONSHIP WITH HUSBAND	.028	−.125	.011

*p < .05
**p < .01
***p < .0005

anxious. The negative correlation between feeling depressed and functional status also was statistically significant during each trimester ($p < .05$); those women who reported feeling depressed performed their usual activities at a lower level throughout pregnancy than did the women who did not report feeling depressed.

Just a few (4%) women stated that they were hindered in the performance of their usual activities by various negative psychological symptoms. One woman explained that she was hindered because she "worried about her baby." Another noted that she was hindered because she had feelings of "anxiety about how things would turn out."

Other women commented that they were hindered because they felt moody or depressed at times. One of those woman stated: "I am an emotional person anyway, and so those hormones really did [hinder my activities]. I would get depressed and think about things that at the time seemed important—like money, what are we going to do, how are we going to [manage] financial[ly]." Another commented that she was hindered because she "was pretty depressed about being pregnant. I think I should have been happier—it was a good experience."

Still another women noted that she was hindered by a feeling of "indifference to my pregnancy." One other woman noted that because her "head was like absent-mindedness," she could not always perform her usual activities.

The positive correlation between feeling better than usual and functional status was statistically significant only in the first trimester ($p < .01$). The women who reported feeling better than usual at the beginning of pregnancy performed their usual activities at a higher level than those who did not report feeling better than usual at that time.

Almost one fifth (18%) of the women indicated that attitude was a key factor in helping them to continue their usual activities during pregnancy. One woman, for example, simply stated: "My general attitude [helped]." A feeling of self-determination was helpful for some women. One woman cited her "self determination" as helpful, and another commented that she thought, "I can do this." Another woman stated, "I was determined to do things until the end." Similarly, another women commented, "My attitude [helped]. I would never expect not to do my thing or say, 'Well, I am pregnant, I can't do it.' " A sense of humor also was helpful, as documented by a woman who stated, "Keeping my sense of humor [was helpful]; that was, without a doubt, the one thing that holds your sanity together."

Two women noted that they pampered themselves. One woman explained that she did "certain things for myself that were psychological, like buying nice soaps, getting my hair cut, and that sort of thing." The other noted that she did not "feel bad about taking naps in the middle of the day."

Changes in PNSQ Psychosocial Health Variables

Examination of the PNSQ scores for variables representing psychosocial health (the woman's acceptance of her pregnancy; her identification of a motherhood role; her feelings regarding preparation for labor; her fear of pain, helplessness, and loss of control during labor; and her concern for the well-being of herself and her baby) revealed relatively positive evaluations, as well as some changes across the three trimesters of pregnancy (Table 4.1). The woman's acceptance of her pregnancy increased from the first to the second trimester ($p < .0005$); no change in acceptance was evident from the second to the third trimester. In addition, the woman's feelings regarding preparation for labor become more positive in the third trimester, when compared with the second trimester ($p < .0005$); there was no change from the first to the second trimester. Although there was an overall statistically significant change in the woman's identification of a motherhood role ($p = .04$), no statistically significant changes were evident from trimester to trimester. No evidence of changes was found for the woman's fear of pain, helplessness, and loss of control during labor, or for her concern for the well-being of herself and her baby.

Some women's comments at six months postpartum indicated their acceptance of the pregnancy and confidence in themselves. For example, one woman stated:

> I think the fact that I knew what was happening with the pregnancy all along, and I felt very much that I understood the baby; now that he is six months old and I see how he has turned out, it is the same as I thought when he was in utero. And I think the fact that I felt very close to him in utero made me very confident in keeping doing everything that I was doing. I felt very sure and understood when he was resting [and when he was active]; I think I understood what made him do what he did.

PNSQ Psychosocial Health Variables and Functional Status

The correlations between the PNSQ psychosocial health variables and functional status were of relatively low magnitude (Table 4.2). Although all of the signs of the correlations are negative, the relations are positive because lower PSNQ scores indicate positive evaluations (see Appendix). The correlations between the woman's acceptance of pregnancy ($p < .0005$), as well as her concern for the well-being of herself and her baby ($p < .01$), and functional status were statistically significant during each trimester. Thus, a higher level of performance of usual activities was associated with the woman's greater acceptance of pregnancy and less concern about her own and her baby's well-being.

The correlation between the woman's fear of pain, helplessness, and loss of control during labor and functional status was statistically significant for all three trimesters ($p < .01$), such that a higher level of performance of usual activities was associated with less fear throughout pregnancy. The correlation between the woman's feelings of preparation for labor and functional status was statistically significant for the first and third trimesters only ($p < .05$), indicating that a higher level of functional status was associated with feelings of greater preparation for labor at those times. Finally, the correlation between the woman's identification of a motherhood role and functional status was statistically significant only in the second trimester ($p < .05$), indicating that a higher level of performance of usual activities was associated with greater identification with the role of motherhood only at that time.

Changes in Family Relationships

Examination of the PNSQ scores for variables representing family relationships revealed relatively positive evaluations, as well as evidence of a change in the woman's relationship with her husband but not in her relationship with her mother (Table 4.1). The woman's relationship with her husband was more positive in the first trimester than in the second ($p < .0005$); no change was evident from the second to the third trimester.

Family Relationships and Functional Status

The correlations between the PNSQ family relationships variables—relationship with mother and relationship with husband—and functional status were exceptionally low in magnitude (Table 4.2). There was no evidence of an association between either family relationships variable and functional status at any time during the pregnancy ($p >$ .05). Yet more than one quarter of the women told us that their husband (24%) or mother (4%) helped them to continue their usual activities throughout the pregnancy. When asked what helped them to continue their usual activities, some women simply answered, "My husband." More elaborate representative comments are as follows:

> My husband was very helpful. He took over a lot of household chores so that I could keep up with my studies.

> My husband took care of my son a lot more, especially when I was sick and felt lousy. He was really helpful in getting me through that period.

> My husband was my encouragement. I wanted to lay down and sleep all the time. He got me going.

Two women who noted that their mothers were particularly helpful provided global comments: "Having my mom to help out." and "The help from my mom." Elaborating, another woman stated: "My mother was retired, and she was able to help me with things that I couldn't do when I was sick." Still another woman explained, "Having my mother watch my daughter was a lot less stressful than with a baby sitter or day care when I worked two days a week."

CONCLUSION

Examination of women's psychosocial health, family relationships, and functional status revealed some changes over the three trimesters of pregnancy. As expected from our Theory of Adaptation During Childbearing and in keeping with the Roy Adaptation Model, changes occurred in the variables representing the self-concept and interdependence modes as the focal stimulus of pregnancy progressed. Moreover, the correlations between the variables representing the Roy Adaptation Model self-concept and role function response modes indicate that these modes are interrelated components of adaptation during pregnancy. This finding is in keeping with the results of a meta-analysis of the interrelation between these two Roy Adaptation Model response modes (Chiou, 2000). There was, however, no evidence of an interrelationship between the interdependence mode, represented by family relationships variables, and the role function mode, represented by functional status, in our study. That finding conflicts with the results of Chiou's (2000) meta-analysis; she found evidence of an association between variables representing the role function and interdependence modes across four studies.

Our results add to existing knowledge about the psychosocial health and family relationships variables included in the PNSQ and also point to the need for continued research to further determine the stability of results across studies. Some of our findings are similar to those of the few longitudinal studies employing the PNSQ. Our finding of an increase in the woman's acceptance of pregnancy from the first to the second trimester is similar to Hall's (1991) finding of an increase in that variable from the second to the third trimester, as well as to Randell's (1988) and Lederman, Harrison, and Worsham's (1993, 1994) finding of an increase from the first to the third trimester. Moreover, our finding of an increase in the woman's feelings of preparation for labor from the second to the third trimester replicates Hall's (1991) data and is similar to Lederman, Harrison, and Worsham's (1993, 1994) finding of an increase from the first to the third trimester.

Our study results are not completely in keeping with the other longitudinal studies in which the PNSQ was used. Our finding of no changes in women's identification of a motherhood role conflicts with Randell's (1988) finding of an increase in that variable from the first to the third trimester of pregnancy. Furthermore, our finding of no changes in fears about labor from trimester to trimester conflicts with other investigators' findings of decreases in labor fears from the first to the second trimester (Hall, 1991) and from the second to the third trimester (Lederman, Harrison, & Worsham, 1993, 1994). In addition, our finding of no changes in the woman's concern for the well-being of herself and her baby conflicts with Lederman, Harrison, and Worsham's (1993, 1994) finding of an decrease in concern from the second to the third trimester.

Our findings for the PNSQ family relationships variables add to the confusion about whether the woman's relationships with her mother and her husband change. Our finding of no changes in the woman's evaluation of her relationship with her mother conflicts with Randell's (1988) finding of improvement in the relationship with mother from the first to the third trimester, but is in keeping with Hall's (1991) and Lederman, Harrison, and Worsham's (1993, 1994) findings of no evidence of changes.

Furthermore, our finding of a decrease in the woman's evaluation of her relationship with her husband from the first to the second trimester followed by an slight increase from the second to the third trimester conflicts with Hall's (1991) and Lederman, Harrison, and Worsham's (1993, 1994) findings of no change from trimester to trimester. Moreover, our finding of fluctuation from trimester to trimester conflicts with Richardson's (1981) finding of change in the woman's relationship with her husband from early to midpregnancy, followed by stability until the end of the pregnancy.

Inasmuch as many women attend childbirth classes and also begin to discuss their birth plans with health care professionals during the third trimester of pregnancy, it was not surprising that we found that the women in our study experienced greater feelings of preparation for labor at that time than during the second trimester. Noteworthy, however, is our finding of no changes in the women's fears about labor. Research is needed to determine the effects of childbirth education on their fear of labor.

The correlations between functional status and psychological symptoms and PNSQ variables reported in this chapter extend understanding of the extent to which psychosocial health and family relationships variables influence the woman's performance of her usual activities during pregnancy. Each of the three psychological symptoms and all of the PNSQ variables representing psychosocial health were related to functional status at some time during the pregnancy (Table 4.2).

The link between psychological symptoms and functional status requires further exploration. We were able to determine only that there was a negative relation between feeling anxious and functional status, and between feeling depressed and functional status. Future research should examine three possible relationships: (1) that limitations in the woman's performance of usual activities engender anxiety and depression; (2) that feelings of anxiety and depression lead to decreased performance of usual activities; or (3) that the relation is reciprocal. If it is determined that the relation is, indeed, reciprocal, additional research will be needed to determine the starting point, as well as other variables that may act as a catalyst, such as the occurrence of certain physical symptoms (see chapter 2).

Similarly, the link between the PSNQ psychosocial health variables and functional status requires exploration. We were able to uncover only positive relations. As with psychological symptoms, the direction of the relationship and whether it is reciprocal should be the topic of a future study.

In contrast to the findings for functional status and the psychosocial health variables, neither of the PNSQ variables representing family relationships was related to functional status at any time during the pregnancy. Evidently, a woman's relationships with her family members do not influence her performance of usual activities while she is pregnant. Indeed, in light of Samarel, Fawcett, and Tulman's (1997) finding of no relation between the quality of a woman's relationship with her significant other and functional status during the period of treatment for breast cancer, it may be that relationships with significant others have no bearing on functioning at any time.

REFERENCES

Affonso, D. D., Liu-Chiang, C-Y., & Mayberry, L. J. (1999). Worry: Conceptual dimensions and relevance to childbearing women. *Health Care for Women International, 20,* 227–236.

Affonso, D. D., Lovett, S., Paul, S. M., & Sheptak, S. (1990). A standardized interview that differentiates pregnancy and postpartum symptoms from perinatal clinical depression. *Birth, 17,* 121–130.

Affonso, D. D., Lovett, S., Paul, S. M., Sheptak, S., Nussbaum, R., Newman, L., & Johnson, B. (1992). Dysphoric distress in childbearing women. *Journal of Perinatology, 12,* 325–332.

Affonso, D., Mayberry, L., Lovett, S., Paul, S., Johnson, B., Nussbaum, R., & Newman, L. (1993). Pregnancy and postpartum depressive symptoms. *Journal of Women's Health, 2,* 157–164.

Arizmendi, T. G., & Affonso, D. D. (1987). Stressful events related to pregnancy and postpartum. *Journal of Psychosomatic Research, 31,* 743–756.

Behrenz, K. M., & Monga, M. (1999). Fatigue in pregnancy: A comparative study. *American Journal of Perinatology, 16,* 185–188.

Buckwalter, J. G., Stanczyk, F. Z., McCleary, C. A., Bluestein, B. W., Buckwalter, D. K., Rankin, K. P., Chang, L., & Goodwin, T. M. (1999). Pregnancy, the postpartum, and steroid hormones: Effects on cognition and mood. *Psychoneuroendocrinology, 24,* 69–84.

Chiou, C-P. (2000). A meta-analysis of the interrelationships between the modes in Roy's adaptation model. *Nursing Science Quarterly, 13,* 252–258.

Condon, J. T. (1987). Psychological and physical symptoms during pregnancy: A comparison of male and female expectant parents. *Journal of Reproductive and Infant Psychology, 5,* 207–219.

Cunningham, F. G., MacDonald, P. C., & Gant, N. F. (1997). *William's obstetrics* (20th ed.). Stamford, CT: Appleton & Lange.

Drake, M. L., Verhulst, D., & Fawcett, J. (1988). Physical and psychological symptoms experienced by Canadian women and their husbands during pregnancy and the postpartum. *Journal of Advanced Nursing, 13,* 436–440.

Fawcett, J., & York, R. (1986). Spouses' physical and psychological symptoms during pregnancy and the postpartum. *Nursing Research, 35,* 144–148.

Fawcett, J., & York, R. (1987). Spouses' strength of identification and reports of symptoms during pregnancy and the postpartum. *Florida Nursing Review, 2*(2), 1–10.

Gjerdingen, D. K., Froberg, D. G., & Kochevar, L. (1991). Changes in women's mental and physical health from pregnancy through six months postpartum. *Journal of Family Practice, 32*(2), 1–6.

Glazer, G. (1980). Anxiety levels and concerns among pregnant women. *Research in Nursing and Health, 3,* 107–113.

Gotlib, I. H., Wiffen, V. E., Mount, J. H., Milne, K., & Cordy, N. I. (1989). Prevalence rates and demographic characteristics associated with depression in pregnancy and the postpartum. *Journal of Consulting and Clinical Psychology, 57,* 269–274.

Gottesman, M. M. (1992). Maternal adaptation to pregnancy among adult early, middle, and late childbearers: Similarities and differences. *Maternal-Child Nursing Journal, 20,* 93–110.

Grush, L. R., & Cohen, L. S. (1998). Treatment of depression during pregnancy: Balancing the risks. *Harvard Review of Psychiatry, 6,* 105–109.

Haglund, L. J., & Britton, J. R. (1998). The perinatal assessment of psychosocial risk. *Clinics in Perinatology, 25,* 417–452.

Hall, S. L. (1991). *The development of self-concept during the three trimesters of pregnancy.* Unpublished doctoral dissertation, University of Texas, Austin.

Halman, L. J., Oakley, D., & Lederman, R. (1995). Adaptation to pregnancy and motherhood among subfecund and fecund primiparous women. *Maternal-Child Nursing Journal, 23,* 90–100.

Hobbs, D. F. (1965). Parenthood as crisis: A third study. *Journal of Marriage and the Family, 27,* 367–378.

Hobbs, D. F., & Cole, S. P. (1976). Transition to parenthood: A decade replication. *Journal of Marriage and the Family, 38,* 723–731.

Hughes, P. M., Turton, P., & Evans, C. D. H. (1999). Stillbirth as a risk factor for depression and anxiety in the subsequent pregnancy: Cohort study. *British Medical Journal, 318,* 1721–1724.

Kaplan, B. J. (1986). A psychobiological review of depression during pregnancy. *Psychology of Women Quarterly, 10,* 35–48.

Lederman, R. P. (1984). Anxiety and conflict in pregnancy: Relationship to maternal health status. In H. H. Werley & J. J. Fitzpatrick (Eds.), *Annual review of nursing research* (Vol. 2, pp. 27–61). New York: Springer Publishing.

Lederman, R. P. (1986). Maternal anxiety in pregnancy: Relationship to fetal and newborn health status. In H. H. Werley, J. J. Fitzpatrick, & R. L. Taunton (Eds.), *Annual review of nursing research* (Vol. 4, pp. 3–19). New York: Springer Publishing.

Lederman, R. P. (1996). *Psychosocial adaptation in pregnancy: Assessment of seven dimensions of maternal development* (2nd ed.). New York: Springer Publishing.

Lederman, R. P., Harrison, J., & Worsham, S. (1993, June). *Psychosocial predictors of pregnancy adaptation and outcome in a multicultural, low-income population.* Paper presented at the NAACOG Conference, Minneapolis, MN.

Lederman, R. P., Harrison, J., & Worsham, S. (1994). Maternal prenatal developmental differences in three ethnic groups. In D. Turk (Ed.), *Proceedings of the*

Society of Behavioral Medicine Fifteenth Annual Scientific Sessions (Vol. 16, Suppl.). Boston: Society of Behavioral Medicine.

Lederman, R. P., & Lederman, E. (1996). Methods of assessment. In R. P. Lederman, *Psychosocial adaptation in pregnancy: Assessment of seven dimensions of maternal development* (2nd ed., pp. 274–308). New York: Springer Publishing.

Lederman, R. P., & Miller, D. S. (1998). Adaptation to pregnancy in three different ethnic groups: Latin-American, African-American, and Anglo-American. *Canadian Journal of Nursing Research, 30*(3), 37–51.

Leifer, M. (1980). *Psychological effects of motherhood: A study of first pregnancy.* New York: Praeger.

Lips, H. M. (1985). A longitudinal study of the reporting of emotional and somatic symptoms during and after pregnancy. *Social Science and Medicine, 21,* 631–640.

Newton, N. (1955). *Maternal emotions: A study of women's feelings toward menstruation, pregnancy, childbirth, breast feeding, infant care, and other aspects of their femininity.* New York: Paul B. Hoeber.

O'Hara, M. W. (1986). Social support, life events, and depression during pregnancy and the puerperium. *Archives of General Psychiatry, 43,* 569–573.

Randell, B. P. (1988). *Older primiparous women: The evolution of maternal self-perception within the context of mother-daughter and spousal relationships.* Unpublished doctoral dissertation, University of California, San Francisco.

Reading, A. E. (1983). The influence of maternal anxiety on the course and outcome of pregnancy: A review. *Health Psychology, 2,* 187–202.

Reeder, S. J., Martin, L. L., & Koniak-Griffin, D. (1997). *Maternity nursing: Family, newborn, and women's health care* (18th ed.). Philadelphia: Lippincott-Raven.

Richardson, P. (1981). Women's perceptions of their important dyadic relationships during pregnancy. *Maternal Child Nursing Journal, 10,* 159–174.

Rini, C. K., Dunkel-Schetter, C., Wadhwa, P. D., & Sandman, C. A. (1999). Psychological adaptation and birth outcomes: The role of personal resources, stress, and sociocultural context in pregnancy. *Health Psychology, 18,* 333–345.

Samarel, N., Fawcett, J., & Tulman, L. (1997). Effect of support groups with coaching on adaptation to early stage breast cancer. *Research in Nursing and Health, 20,* 15–26.

Schroeder-Zwelling, E. (1988). The pregnancy experience. In F. H. Nichols & S. S. Humenick, *Childbirth education: Practice, research and theory* (pp. 37–51). Philadelphia: Saunders.

Stark, M. A. (1997). Psychosocial adjustment during pregnancy: The experience of mature gravidas. *Journal of Obstetrical, Gynecological, and Neonatal Nursing, 26,* 206–211.

Teixeira, J. M. A., Fisk, N. M., & Glover, V. (1999). Association between maternal anxiety in pregnancy and increased uterine artery resistance index: Cohort based study. *British Medical Journal, 318,* 153–157.

Uddenberg, N., Fagerström, C. F., & Hakanson-Zaunders, M. (1976). Reproductive conflicts, mental symptoms during pregnancy and time in labour. *Journal of Psychosomatic Research, 20,* 575–581.

Walker, L. O., Cooney, A. T., & Riggs, M. W. (1999). Psychosocial and demographic factors related to health behaviors in the 1st trimester. *Journal of Obstetric, Gynecologic, and Neonatal Nursing, 28,* 606–614.

White, J. M. (1992). Marital status and well-being in Canada. *Journal of Family Issues, 13,* 390–401.

Zajicek, E., & Wolkind, S. (1978). Emotional difficulties in married women during and after first pregnancy. *British Journal of Medical Psychology, 51,* 379–385.

Zachariah, R. (1994a). Maternal-fetal attachment: Influence of mother-daughter and husband-wife relationships. *Research in Nursing and Health, 17,* 37–44.

Zachariah, R. (1994b). Mother-daughter and husband-wife attachment as predictors of psychological well-being during pregnancy. *Clinical Nursing Research, 3,* 371–392.

Part III

ADAPTATION AFTER DELIVERY

5

Physical Health and Functional Status During the Postpartum

The first few weeks and months after childbirth are a time of considerable adaptation in a woman's life. Classic studies have focused almost exclusively on the process of maternal role attainment and factors that influence transition to the maternal role (Mercer, 1986, 1995; Rubin, 1984). Our previous study extended the research to the investigation of changes in, and variables associated with, functional status during the first six months following childbirth (Tulman, Fawcett, Groblewski, & Silverman, 1990). In this chapter, we present the part of our Theory of Adaptation During Childbearing dealing with physical health and functional status during the first six months of the postpartum (Figures 5.1 and 5.2). In keeping with the Roy Adaptation Model and the available evidence from the literature, we proposed that functional status, physical energy, and physical symptoms would change throughout the first six months postpartum (Figure 5.2 [A]). We also proposed that physical energy and physical symptoms would be related to functional status at three weeks, six weeks, three months, and six months postpartum (Figure 5.2 [B]).

The research we report in this chapter represents a replication and extension of our previous study (Tulman, Fawcett, Groblewski, & Silverman, 1990). Here, we extend our conceptualization of physical health from physical energy to both physical energy and common physical symptoms. We also explored the influence of type of delivery, medical restrictions, and minor intrapartal, postpartal, and neonatal complications on functional status.

ROLE THEORY AND FUNCTIONAL STATUS

As explained in chapter 2, role theory suggests that changes may occur in the performance of various activities during the childbearing period when the maternal role is being attained or readjusted to accommodate the new infant. Accordingly, we proposed that functional status changes

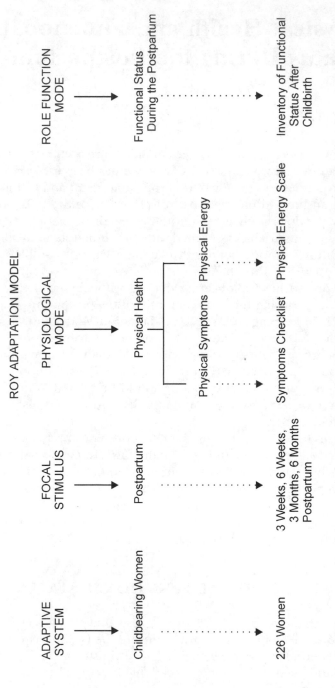

FIGURE 5.1 Linkages between the Roy Adaptation Model, physical health and functional status, and study variables and measures.

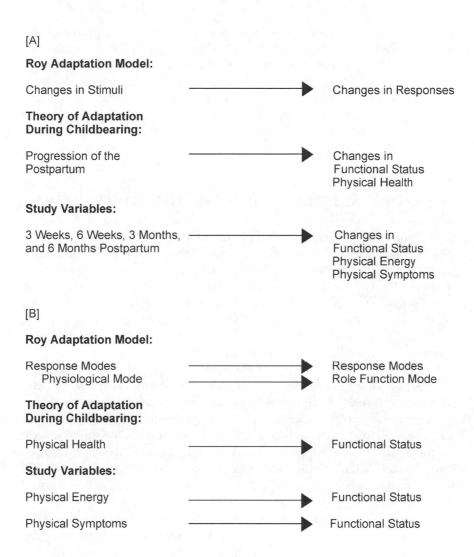

[A]

Roy Adaptation Model:

Changes in Stimuli ⟶ Changes in Responses

Theory of Adaptation During Childbearing:

Progression of the Postpartum ⟶ Changes in Functional Status Physical Health

Study Variables:

3 Weeks, 6 Weeks, 3 Months, and 6 Months Postpartum ⟶ Changes in Functional Status Physical Energy Physical Symptoms

[B]

Roy Adaptation Model:

Response Modes ⟶ Response Modes
   Physiological Mode ⟶ Role Function Mode

Theory of Adaptation During Childbearing:

Physical Health ⟶ Functional Status

Study Variables:

Physical Energy ⟶ Functional Status

Physical Symptoms ⟶ Functional Status

FIGURE 5.2 Diagrams of propositions of the Roy Adaptation Model, the Theory of Adaptation During Childbearing, and study variables: Functional status and physical health during the postpartum.

not only during pregnancy but also during the first six months of the postpartum as the woman actively takes on the role of mother. During that time, the woman may give up some of her usual activities or change the extent to which she performs those activities as she adds the activities associated with infant care. We have defined postpartum functional status as the extent to which the woman resumes her usual personal care, household, social and community, child care, occupational, and educational activities, and assumes infant care responsibilities.

FUNCTIONAL STATUS DURING THE POSTPARTUM

Textbooks imply that full recovery of all areas of functional status proba- bly occurs simultaneously with healing of the reproductive organs by six weeks following delivery (Cunningham, MacDonald, & Gant, 1997; Reeder, Martin, & Koniak-Griffin, 1997). Yet there is some evidence that functional status continues to change after the first six postpartum weeks. Hiser (1987) found that during the second postpartum week, multiparas were especially concerned about their ability to meet family members' needs, finding time for themselves, taking effective and safe care of their infants, and being good mothers. Fishbein and Burggraf (1998), who used the *Inventory of Functional Status After Childbirth* (IFSAC) (Fawcett, Tulman, & Myers, 1988) to measure activities, reported that at one month postpartum, most of the 92 women in their study had assumed responsibility for infant care activities and had resumed several of their usual household activities. Most of the women also had resumed their usual social activities with family members and friends, but few had resumed usual community-based activities. Very few of the women had resumed full performance of their personal care activities.

Gruis (1977) found that the major concerns of both primiparas and multiparas at one month after delivery included coordinating the multiple demands of household, infant, and family responsibilities, as well as finding time for personal activities and exercise. Primiparas were especially concerned about infant care, whereas multiparas were concerned about the effects of a new child on the family. A replication of Gruis's study revealed similar findings for a group of primiparous and multiparous mothers from whom data were collected at three weeks to two months after delivery (Harrison & Hicks, 1983). The findings of an earlier study (Larsen, 1966) revealed that during the first three months postpartum, primiparas and multiparas reported a number of stresses, including difficulty in adjusting to the needs of the baby and other children, difficulty with housework and routines, and worry over ability to cope with family needs. Mothers with three children noted that adjusting to the needs of a baby and two older children was particularly difficult.

Sampselle and colleagues (1999) reported that just 35% of the 1,003 women in their study engaged in vigorous physical activities at six weeks after delivery. More than one half (55%) of the women indicated that their current level of activity was less than usual; just 29% indicated that their current activity level was the same as usual, and only 16% indicated that their current activity level was greater than usual. Less than one half of the women indicated that they were performing activities they regarded as fun, such as hobbies (48%), socializing (47%), sports (47%), and entertainment (39%).

McVeigh (1997a), who administered the IFSAC to 132 Australian women at six weeks postpartum, reported that none of the women had resumed full functional status for personal care activities. Few women had resumed full functional status in the areas of social and community activities (8%) or household activities (17%). Slightly less than one half (47%) had assumed full functional status for infant care activities. Less than one fifth (18%) of the 17 women who had returned to work had resumed overall full functional status.

Koenigseder (1991) reported statistically significant improvements in functional status, as measured by the IFSAC, from Day 3 to Day 7 to Day 14 to Day 21 of the postpartum in sample of 33 women who were followed from Day 3 to Day 42 of the postpartum. Only two thirds (67%) of the women had fully resumed their usual levels of household and social and community activities, and just 6% had resumed their usual level of personal care activities by Day 42 (i.e., six weeks postpartum). One fifth (21%) of the women had not fully assumed their desired or required level of infant care activities by that time.

Smith-Hanrahan and Deblois (1995) reported an improvement in functional status, as measured by the IFSAC, from the first to the sixth postpartum week for 81 women. More specifically, they found that the total IFSAC score increased, as did the scores for personal care activities, household activities, and social and community activities ($p < .001$). There was, however, no evidence of a change in the score for infant care activities.

Our own earlier research supports our contention that women require far more than six weeks to return to their usual activities following childbirth (Tulman, Fawcett, Groblewski, & Silverman, 1990). Our findings revealed that functional status, as measured by the IFSAC, improved progressively between three and six weeks ($p < .0005$) and between six weeks and three months ($p < .0005$); however, no changes in scores were evident between three and six months ($p = .148$). Yet, even by six months postpartum, 83% of the 87 women in our study had not resumed their usual full level of personal care activities, 20% had not resumed their full level of household activities, and 30% had not fully resumed their social and community activities. Moreover, 60% of those women who had returned to work or school by six months following delivery had not fully resumed their usual level of occupational or educational activities.

McVeigh (1998) reported similar findings from her longitudinal study of 173 Australian women who completed the IFSAC at six weeks, three months, and six months postpartum. She found increases in scores for the household activities ($p = .0001$) and social and community activities ($p = .0001$) IFSAC subscales from six weeks to three months and from three months to six months after delivery. The score for the personal care activities subscale increased only from six weeks to three months ($p = .0006$). No changes were noted in the scores for the infant care activities and occupational activities subscales throughout the study period. None of the women had achieved full functional status in all activities by six months postpartum. Almost 60% had not fully resumed their usual household activities, 70% had not fully resumed their usual social and community activities, and more than 75% of the 26 women who had returned to work had not fully resumed their usual occupational activities.

PHYSICAL HEALTH DURING THE POSTPARTUM

Physical Energy

Women frequently experience a deficit in physical energy during the postpartum. Reasons given for that deficit include the poor quality of sleep during the last few weeks of pregnancy, the typically exhausting work of childbirth, and the lack of rest in the first few days of the postpartum that is a direct result of early hospital discharge and the subsequent immediate assumption of all infant care activities (Reeder, Martin, & Koniak-Griffin, 1997).

As we explained in chapter 2, physical energy is conceptually related to fatigue. Fatigue, or physical tiredness, which is an exceptionally common concern of new mothers (Gardner, 1991; Gruis, 1977; Harrison & Hicks, 1983; Pugh, Milligan, Parks, Lenz, & Kitzman, 1999; Ruchala & Halstead, 1994), leads to loss of energy (Campbell, 1986). Smith-Hanrahan and Deblois (1995) found that the level of fatigue varies during the early postpartum weeks, from 95% of the 81 women reporting fatigue at the time of hospital discharge (range = 26–81 hours following delivery), to 96% at one week postpartum, to 86% at six weeks postpartum.

Troy and Dalgas-Pelish (1997) found no statistically significant differences in either morning or evening fatigue scores in a group of 36 women they followed for the first six postpartum weeks. The 30 women who participated in Lee and Zaffke's (1999) longitudinal study reported, on average, higher levels of fatigue during the postpartum than at any time during pregnancy; there was, however, no statistically significant difference in the level of fatigue from one to three months postpartum.

More relevant to our research are studies of energy level during the postpartum. There was no evidence of a statistically significant change in either the morning or evening energy scores throughout the first six postpartum weeks for the women in Troy and Dalgas-Pelish's (1997) study. The women in Lee and Zaffke's (1999) study reported less energy during the first and third postpartum months than during the second and third trimesters of pregnancy. We found that only 51% of the 70 women in our early retrospective study reported they had regained their usual level of physical energy by the end of the sixth postpartum week (Tulman & Fawcett, 1988). In a later study, we found that only 25% of the women had regained their usual level of physical energy by three weeks postpartum, only 54% by six weeks, 76% by three months, and 89% by six months postpartum (Tulman, Fawcett, Groblewski, & Silverman, 1990).

Physical Energy and Functional Status

Some evidence supports the assertion that postpartum functional status is influenced by fatigue or physical energy. Data from interviews of 50 women at 10 to 14 days postpartum revealed that fatigue adversely affected performance of household activities and social activities (Ruchala & Halstead, 1994). McVeigh (1997a) found that women who were dissatisfied with their level of stamina and well-being had a lower level of functional status in the areas of household, personal care, and social and community activities than women who were satisfied with their stamina and well-being level.

Campbell (1986) reported that loss of energy left new mothers feeling so drained that they did not perform their usual household activities. Moreover, the findings of one of our earlier studies linked level of physical energy with performance of household activities and social and community activities at six weeks postpartum (Tulman & Fawcett, 1988). Yet several women in that study commented that they had resumed their usual activities before they had regained their usual level of physical energy. They attributed the early resumption of activities to family obligations, financial constraints, or their own need to appear to have recovered.

The findings of our earlier study revealed that level of physical energy also was significantly associated with functional status at three weeks, six weeks, and six months postpartum (Tulman, Fawcett, Groblewski, & Silverman, 1990). More specifically, a higher level of physical energy was associated with higher levels of performance of household, social and community, and personal care activities at three weeks, six weeks, and six months postpartum. A higher level of physical energy also was associated with higher levels of performance of infant care activities, but only at six months postpartum.

Physical Symptoms

Women experience a variety of physical symptoms during the postpartum. A review of the literature yielded an extensive list of symptoms, including discomfort from an episiotomy or Caesarean section incision, uterine cramps, breast engorgement or infection, nipple irritation, poor appetite, fatigue, anemia, thyroid disorders, hot flashes, increased sweating, dizziness, acne, sleep disturbances, carpal tunnel syndrome, hand numbness or tingling, excessive vaginal bleeding, gynecological infections, urological infections, stress incontinence, hemorrhoids, constipation, and sexual concerns (Gjerdingen, Froberg, Chaloner, & McGovern, 1993; Gjerdingen, Froberg, & Fontaine, 1990). In addition, Kristiansson and colleagues (1996) reported that almost 10% of the 200 women in their study reported back pain after delivery.

Empirical evidence indicates that some changes occur in the prevalence of specific physical symptoms experienced as the time since delivery progresses. For example, at two weeks after delivery, women tend to experience discomfort from sutures (Fishbein & Burggraf, 1998; Ruchala & Halstead, 1994) and hemorrhoids (Ruchala & Halstead, 1994), whereas at six weeks after delivery, feelings of tiredness and constipation frequently are experienced (Fawcett & York, 1986). At about eight weeks postpartum, a group of 72 women reported experiencing, on average, four physical problems. The wide variety of problems involved the genitourinary system (57%); head, eyes, ears, and/or nose (54%); digestive system (47%); musculoskeletal system (32%); respiratory system (26%); skin and/or hair (26%); breasts (15%); circulatory system (11%); and blood and/or endocrine glands (7%) (Gjerdingen & Froberg, 1991). Gjerdingen and colleagues (1993) reported that poor appetite, hand numbness, increased sweating, hot flashes, fatigue, constipation, hemorrhoids, vaginal discomfort, and dizziness all were more prevalent at one month after delivery than at three or six months.

Some evidence indicates that the number of physical symptoms actually increases, rather than decreases, during the postpartum. Mercer's (1995) review of the literature revealed that women report more physical health problems as the postpartum progresses. Specific symptoms include headaches, respiratory infections, fatigue, gastrointestinal problems, and gynecological problems. Gjerdingen, Froberg, and Kochevar (1991) found that women experienced more days of illness at six months postpartum than they had at six weeks or three months after delivery. Despite the increase in illness days, Gjerdingen and colleagues (1993) reported that a wide variety of physical symptoms decreased progressively throughout the first postpartum year. The exceptions were respiratory symptoms, which increased after the first postpartum month; sexual symptoms, which increased from one to three months postpartum; and hair loss, which increased progressively from one to six months after delivery.

Physical Symptoms and Functional Status

No studies of a direct link between physical symptoms and functional status during the postpartum were located. However, McVeigh (1997b) found that Australian women who experienced personal illness had a lower level of performance of social and community activities, as measured by the IFSAC, than did women who did not experience illness.

In addition, Brown (1987) reported that women who were planning to return to work within the year after delivery were less likely to report somatic or psychological symptoms than women who did not plan to resume employment.

Type of Delivery and Functional Status

Our earlier research revealed that type of delivery was related to functional status, such that women who had a vaginal delivery had a higher level of functional status in household, social and community, and personal care activities at three weeks postpartum than women who had a Caesarean delivery. This relation was not, however, evident at six weeks, three months, or six months postpartum (Tulman, Fawcett, Groblewski, & Silverman, 1990). Similarly, Fawcett (1991) found no evidence of a relation between type of delivery and functional status at six weeks postpartum.

Medical Restrictions and Functional Status

Our earlier research revealed no evidence of an association between medical restrictions, in the form of advice the woman reported she received from her physician or nurse-midwife to restrict her activities, and functional status (Tulman, Fawcett, Groblewski, & Silverman, 1990). No other studies were located.

Complications and Functional Status

The findings of one of our earlier studies indicated that women who experienced either a maternal or a neonatal complication were significantly less likely to resume employment after delivery than women who did not experience a complication (Tulman & Fawcett, 1988). In contrast, the data from a later study revealed no evidence of a relation between minor intrapartal, postpartal, or neonatal complications and functional status (Tulman, Fawcett, Groblewski, & Silverman, 1990).

THE RESULTS OF OUR STUDY

We examined the data from the 226 women who participated in our study throughout the postpartum for changes in overall and specific areas of functional status, and in physical energy and physical symptoms (see Table 5.1). We also looked at the correlations between physical energy and functional status and physical symptoms and functional status during the postpartum (Table 5.2). In addition, we present the women's responses to an interview, which we conducted at six months postpartum. They told us a great deal about what helped and hindered their adaptation during the postpartum.

Changes in Functional Status

Overall functional status and functional status in the specific areas of household, child care, and personal care activities changed during the postpartum ($p < .0005$), with progressive increases from three weeks to six weeks to three months to six months after delivery (Table 5.1). Functional status in social and community activities also changed ($p < .0005$), with progressive increases from three weeks to six weeks and from six weeks to three months postpartum. In addition, functional status in infant care activities changed ($p < .0005$), with statistically significant increases from three weeks to six weeks and from three months to six months after delivery.

Functional status in occupational activities for the 41 women who had returned to work by six weeks postpartum increased from that time to three months after delivery. At six months postpartum, those women who had returned to work had a slightly lower but statistically significant level of functional status than those who did not work ($p = .008$). There was no evidence of a relation between return to work and functional status at any other time during the postpartum. Just six of the women were attending school and were, therefore, involved in educational activities during the postpartum. No evidence of a change in functional status in these activities was found.

When women's overall functional status scores were divided into two categories—less than full functional status and full functional status—the percentage of women reporting full functional status changed during the postpartum ($p < .0005$), with a progressive increase from three weeks (15%) to six weeks (57%) to three months (76%) to six months (85%).

At six months postpartum, one tenth (11%) of the women in our study told us that maintaining their usual activities helped them to adapt to the postpartum experience. One woman stated, "I guess I

TABLE 5.1   Functional Status, Physical Energy, and Physical Symptoms During the Postpartum (*N* = 226)

	3 Weeks Postpartum	6 Weeks Postpartum	3 Months Postpartum	6 Months Postpartum	*p*
FUNCTIONAL STATUS [*M, SD*]**					
Household (*n* = 226)	2.62 (.75)	3.42 (.54)	3.69 (.36)	3.78 (.32)	< .0005[d]
Social/ Community (*n* = 224)	2.59 (.76)	3.16 (.70)	3.51 (.58)	3.53 (.56)	< .0005[a]
Infant Care (*n* = 225)	3.80 (.32)	3.88 (.26)	3.88 (.28)	3.93 (.22)	< .0005[c]
Child Care (*n* = 140)	3.02 (.68)	3.57 (.46)	3.76 (.32)	3.86 (.24)	< .0005[d]
Personal Care (*n* = 225)	2.97 (.45)	3.37 (.33)	3.53 (.31)	3.60 (.29)	< .0005[d]
Occupational[e] (*n* = 41)	—	2.79 (.74)	3.17 (.70)	3.26 (.63)	< .0005[b]
Educational[e] (*n* = 6)	—	3.60 (.36)	3.57 (.51)	3.40 (.38)	.74
Total (*N* = 226)	2.94 (.48)	3.46 (.34)	3.64 (.26)	3.71 (.21)	< .0005[d]
MAINTAIN USUAL LEVEL OF PHYSICAL ENERGY [%]					< .0005[d]
Not At All	9%	2%	1%	1%	
Just Beginning	24%	11%	4%	2%	
Partially	49%	42 %	23%	15%	
Fully	19%	45%	73%	83%	
NUMBER OF PHYSICAL SYMPTOMS [*M, SD*]*	4.58 (2.11)	3.81 (2.23)	3.05 (2.35)	2.58 (2.08)	< .0005[d]

[a]Differences between 3 weeks and 6 weeks and 6 weeks and 3 months statistically significant.
[b]Differences between 6 weeks and 3 months statistically significant.
[c]Differences between 3 weeks and 6 weeks and 3 months and 6 months statistically significant.
[d]Differences between 3 weeks and 6 weeks, 6 weeks and 3 months, and 3 months and 6 months statistically significant.
[e]Too few women had returned to work or school by 3 weeks postpartum for meaningful analysis. Therefore, the analysis is based on the women who were employed or attending school by 6 weeks postpartum.
*Potential range of scores = 0–21 symptoms.
**Potential range of scores = 1.00–4.00, where higher scores indicate greater functional status.

TABLE 5.2 Correlations of Physical Energy and Physical Symptoms with Functional Status During the Postpartum ($N = 226$)

Variable	3 Weeks Postpartum Functional Status	6 Weeks Postpartum Functional Status	3 Months Postpartum Functional Status	6 Months Postpartum Functional Status
PHYSICAL ENERGY	.541***	.507***	.432***	.188*
PHYSICAL SYMPTOMS	−.300***	−.345***	−.305***	−.213**

*$p = .005$
**$p = .001$
***$p < .0005$

didn't sit around. I did things. I kept moving around." Another woman commented that she adapted by "Getting out and trying to go back to how I was, and taking walks and doing stuff like that, how I used to. I don't get to ride my bike anymore but I take walks with [my baby] now that the weather is warm." Still another woman noted, "The thing that helped me the most was that I ran straight up until the day [my baby] was born. And I [was] out the next day at the park. And by five days after [my baby was born], I was running. Running is the way I need to do it."

A few (2%) women noted that postpartum adaptation was hindered by a change in their usual activities. One of those women commented, "We don't have the same life style . . . you don't have as much freedom." Another woman explained, "I haven't gotten back on track. I am not working out like I was before. I am tired a lot. I have become lazy. I want to get back to that because I know that I will feel better. I am taking care of everyone and not paying attention to me."

Changes in Physical Energy

The women's level of physical energy changed during the postpartum ($p < .0005$), with a progressive increase from three weeks to six weeks to three months to six months (Table 5.1). Slightly less than one fifth (19%) of the women reported maintaining their usual level of physical energy at three weeks postpartum; the number increased to slightly more than two fifths (45%) at six weeks postpartum. At three months postpartum, almost three quarters (73%) of the women reported maintaining their usual level of physical energy; the number increased to slightly more than fourth fifths (83%) at six months postpartum.

Physical Energy and Functional Status

The correlations between physical energy and functional status were of moderate magnitude at three weeks, six weeks, and three months postpartum but lower at six months postpartum (Table 5.2). The positive correlation between physical energy and functional status was statistically significant throughout the postpartum ($p < .01$)—women who fully maintained their usual level of physical energy also performed their usual activities at a higher level than did the women who did not maintain or only partially maintained their usual level of physical energy.

Some women (8%) told us that they adapted during the first six postpartum months by conserving their energy. One woman explained, "I made it a priority to sleep; I made that [my] first priority." Another woman commented that she continued to rest throughout the postpartum. Elaborating, she stated, "It is only recently that all of a sudden I feel that I don't need to take my extra nap and I don't need to get to bed early. Whereas all the way up to a couple of weeks ago I was still needing to go to bed early and [was actually] going to bed early."

In contrast, more than one quarter (27%) of the women told us that their postpartum adaptation was hindered by the lack of sleep or sufficient rest, tiredness, fatigue, or lack of usual level of physical energy. One woman explained, "Lack of sleep was the worst of all. [This was because] the baby had his days and nights mixed up for a while. [So, I was] getting up every hour and nursing for an hour and getting a hour [of] sleep and that happened several times. [And,] I cannot nap during the day no matter what." Another women noted that "When you are that tired you don't have the patience. I noticed I took a lot out on my oldest child. He was getting yelled at when [the baby] was upset." Still another women commented, "I still feel tired and I don't feel as energetic as I think that I should feel or as I thought I would." One women linked her lack of energy with breastfeeding. She stated, "I don't have the same energy level because I am nursing him."

Changes in Physical Symptoms

The number of physical symptoms experienced by the women changed during the postpartum ($p < .0005$), with a progressive decrease from three weeks to six weeks to three months to six months (Table 5.1). The most common physical symptoms at three weeks postpartum, in decreasing order of frequency, were feeling tired, feeling less active than usual, increased appetite, backache, and hemorrhoids. At six weeks postpartum, the most common physical symptoms were feeling tired, feeling less active than usual, backache, increased appetite, and hemorrhoids. The most common physical symptoms at three months postpartum were feeling tired, backache, increased appetite, hemorrhoids, and skin irritations. At six months postpartum, the most common physical symptoms were feeling tired, backache, feeling more active than usual, increased appetite, and hemorrhoids.

Physical Symptoms and Functional Status

The correlations between physical symptoms and functional status were of moderate magnitude at three weeks, six weeks, and three months postpartum but were lower at six months postpartum (Table 5.1). The negative correlation between the number of physical symptoms and functional status was statistically significant throughout the postpartum ($p < .005$). Thus, as the number of physical symptoms increased, the women's overall performance of their usual activities decreased.

Almost one tenth (9%) of the women told us that general good health or a lack of physical symptoms helped them to adapt during the postpartum. A representative comment from one woman was: "I took good care of myself during my pregnancy. I ate well and got lots of rest. I am a healthy person."

Type of Delivery, Medical Restrictions, Complications, and Functional Status

We continued to examine the relation between postpartum physical health and functional status by looking at the influence of type of delivery, medical restrictions, and complications. Almost one fifth (18%) of the women had Caesarean deliveries; the remaining four fifths

(82%) had vaginal deliveries, including the few (3%) who had vaginal deliveries after Caesarean (VBAC). We found that women who delivered by Caesarean had lower levels of functional status at three weeks ($p <$ .01) and six months ($p < .05$) than women who experienced vaginal deliveries.

The vast majority (88%) of the women were advised by their health care provider to restrict certain activities immediately after childbirth. The restricted activities included climbing stairs (83%), driving (72%), exercising (63%), housework (57%), walking (30%), going out (19%), bathing or showering (13%), and other activities (26%) such as heavy lifting or sexual intercourse. With one exception, there was no evidence of a relation between a particular restriction and the performance of a related activity at three weeks postpartum. For example, there was no association between restrictions on walking and the IFSAC items for talking walks and walking slowly, both of which are part of the personal care activities subscale. There was, however, an association between restrictions on housework and the IFSAC item for cooking, such that women who had been advised to restrict housework engaged in less cooking than women who had not been so advised ($p = .041$).

One third (33%) of the women experienced complications associated with labor and delivery. Slightly more than one tenth (11%) experienced complications while still in the hospital after delivery. Just over one tenth (12%) experienced childbearing-related complications or other health problems following hospital discharge. Similarly, just over one tenth (12%) of the women reported having complications or other health problems at six weeks postpartum. At three months postpartum, slightly more than one eighth (14%) of the women experienced complications or other health problems. And, at six months postpartum, almost one fifth (18%) of the women reported childbearing complications or other health problems.

When interviewed six months after delivery, more than one fifth (22%) of the women told us that complications or health problems impaired their postpartum adaptation. They cited the following complications and problems: neck pain, back pain, joint and hip pain, discomfort from the episiotomy, hemorrhoids, perineal lacerations, the incision from a Caesarean delivery, nerve damage during delivery, bladder control problems, and a breast infection.

In addition, one fifth (20%) of the women's infants experienced complications while still in the hospital following birth. The percentage of infants who experienced complications progressively decreased, to

15% at three weeks, 10% at six weeks, and 8% at three months, and then increased slightly, to 8% at six months postpartum.

We examined our data to determine the extent to which postpartum complications or other health problems were associated with the women's performance of their usual activities. At three weeks postpartum, woman who experienced complications during labor and delivery ($p <$ .001) or following childbirth while still in the hospital ($p < .05$) performed their usual activities at a lower level than did the women who did not experience complications. Similarly, women whose infants experienced complications while still in the hospital performed their usual activities at a lower level at three weeks postpartum than did the women whose infants did not experience complications ($p < .05$). There was no evidence of a relation between complications or other health problems and functional status at six weeks, three months, or six months postpartum.

CONCLUSION

Women's physical health and functional status changed during the postpartum. As expected from our Theory of Adaptation During Childbearing and in keeping with the Roy Adaptation Model, changes occurred in the variables representing the physiological and role function modes as the focal stimulus of postpartum time progressed. Furthermore, the correlations between the variables representing the Roy Adaptation Model physiological and role function response modes indicated that these modes are interrelated components of adaptation during the postpartum. The finding of relations between those two Roy Adaptation Mode response modes during both pregnancy (see chapter 2) and the postpartum provides considerable support for the results of Chiou's (2000) meta-analytic study of interrelations among the response modes.

Our finding of progressive changes in functional status throughout the first six postpartum months refutes textbook descriptions of full recovery from childbirth by the sixth postpartum week (Cunningham, MacDonald, & Gant, 1997; Reeder, Martin, & Koniak-Griffin, 1997) and adds to the evidence from previous studies indicating that women require more time to resume their usual activities (McVeigh, 1998; Tulman, Fawcett, Groblewski, & Silverman, 1990). More than two fifths (43%) of the women in our study had not attained full functional status at six weeks postpartum, and more than one eighth (15%) had not attained full functional status by six months after delivery.

Although the women in our study reported progressive improvement in their level of physical energy during the first six postpartum months, our findings, coupled with those from previous studies, indicate that women experience a deficit in physical energy for at least six months after childbirth (Lee & Zaffke, 1999; Tulman & Fawcett, 1988; Tulman, Fawcett, Groblewski, & Silverman, 1990). Our finding of a positive correlation between physical energy and functional status, which is in keeping with previous research (Campbell, 1986; McVeigh, 1997a; Ruchala & Halstead, 1994; Tulman & Fawcett, 1988), indicates that deficits in physical energy can affect performance of usual activities.

Our finding of a progressive decline in the number of physical symptoms during the first six postpartum months is consistent with other investigators' findings (Gjerdingen, Froberg, Chaloner, & McGovern, 1993). Gjerdingen, Froberg, and Kochevar's (1991) finding of an increase in days of illness during the postpartum, however, indicates that future studies should be designed to determine the relation between physical symptoms directly associated with childbearing and illness of various etiologies, as well as the meaning of illness to study participants.

Noteworthy is our finding of a change within the list of most frequently reported physical symptoms from feeling *less* active than usual at three and six weeks and three months postpartum, to feeling *more* active than usual at six months. The wording of that item on the *Symptoms Checklist* does not permit us to determine whether the change was due interpretation of the phrase, "as usual," as earlier in the postpartum, prior to delivery, or prior to pregnancy. Clarification of the item is required in future studies.

Our finding of a negative correlation between physical symptoms and functional status throughout the first six postpartum months is consistent with previous studies that linked functional status with illness (McVeigh, 1997b) and health state (Brown, 1987). Taken together, these findings indicate that the occurrence of physical symptoms can affect the woman's performance of her usual activities during the postpartum.

Our findings of a positive correlation between physical energy and functional status and a negative correlation between physical symptoms and functional status during the postpartum are the same as for pregnancy (see chapter 2). Collectively, the consistency in the direction of these correlations calls for a study designed to determine whether a sequential path exists from the occurrence of physical symptoms to a reduction in physical energy to a reduction in the level of functional status. Such a study also should include a measure of functional ability, to determine whether the number of physical symptoms and the level of physical energy affect functional ability, which, in turn, affects functional status (see chapter 2 for a discussion of the distinction between functional ability and functional status).

In keeping with findings from our earlier longitudinal study (Tulman, Fawcett, Groblewski, & Silverman, 1990), we found that type of delivery influenced functional status at three weeks postpartum. In the current study, type of delivery also was related to functional status at six weeks postpartum.

Our finding of an association between complications the women in our study experienced and functional status at three weeks postpartum was limited to those complications directly associated with childbearing or infant complications. These findings, coupled with the finding of no association between any kind of complications or other health problems later in the postpartum, indicate that the circumstances of childbirth do not have a lasting effect on the woman's performance of her usual activities.

Our data yielded empirical evidence of typical restrictions imposed on women by the physician or midwife following delivery. Those restrictions, however, had no major impact on the women's performance of their usual activities during the first few weeks of the postpartum. Future studies should be designed to determine whether the lack of an association between medical restrictions and functional status indicates that women do not follow medical advice following childbirth.

REFERENCES

Brown, M. A. (1987). Employment during pregnancy: Influences on women's health and social support. *Health Care for Women International, 8,* 151–167.

Chiou, C-P. (2000). A meta-analysis of the interrelationships between the modes in Roy's adaptation model. *Nursing Science Quarterly, 13,* 252–258.

Campbell, I. (1986). Postpartum sleep patterns of mother-baby pairs. *Midwifery, 2,* 193–201.

Cunningham, F. G., MacDonald, P. C., & Gant, N. F. (1997). *William's obstetrics* (20th ed.). Stamford, CT: Appleton & Lange.

Fawcett, J. (1991). *Effects of information on adaptation to cesarean birth.* Final report for Grant Number R01-NR01694, National Center for Nursing Research, National Institutes of Health.

Fawcett, J., Tulman, L., & Myers, S. (1988). Development of the Inventory of Functional Status after Childbirth. *Journal of Nurse-Midwifery, 33,* 252–260.

Fawcett, J., & York, R. (1986). Spouses' physical and psychological symptoms during pregnancy and the postpartum. *Nursing Research, 35,* 144–148.

Fishbein, E. G., & Burggraf, E. (1998). Early postpartum discharge: How are mothers managing? *Journal of Obstetric, Gynecologic, and Neonatal Nursing, 27,* 142–148.

Gardner, D. L. (1991). Fatigue in postpartum women. *Applied Nursing Research, 4,* 57–62.

Gjerdingen, D. K., & Froberg, D. G. (1991). The fourth stage of labor: The health of birth mothers and adoptive mothers at 6 weeks postpartum. *Family Medicine, 23,* 29–35.

Gjerdingen, D. K., Froberg, D. G., Chaloner, K. M., & McGovern, P. M. (1993). Changes in women's physical health during the first postpartum year. *Archives of Family Medicine, 2,* 227–283.

Gjerdingen, D. K., Froberg, D. G., & Fontaine, P. (1990). A causal model describing the relationship of women's postpartum health to social support, length of leave, and complications of childbirth. *Women and Health, 16,* 71–87.

Gjerdingen, D. K., Froberg, D. G., & Kochevar, L. (1991). Changes in women's mental and physical health from pregnancy through six months postpartum. *Journal of Family Practice, 32,* 161–166.

Gruis, M. (1977). Beyond maternity: Postpartum concerns of mothers. *MCN, American Journal of Maternal Child Nursing, 2,* 182–188.

Harrison, M. J., & Hicks, S. A. (1983). Postpartum concerns of mothers and their sources of help. *Canadian Journal of Public Health, 74,* 325–328.

Hiser, P. L. (1987). Concerns of multiparas during the second postpartum week. *Journal of Obstetric, Gynecologic, and Neonatal Nursing, 16,* 195–203.

Koenigseder, L. A. (1991). *Patterns of change in primiparas' moods and functional status: An extension of Rubin's nursing model.* Doctoral dissertation, University of Texas at Austin.

Kristiansson, P., Svardsudd, K., & von Schoultz, B. (1996). Back pain during pregnancy: A prospective study. *Spine, 21,* 702–709.

Larsen, V. L. (1966). Stresses of the childbearing year. *American Journal of Public Health, 56,* 32–36.

Lee, K. A., & Zaffke, M. (1999). Longitudinal changes in fatigue and energy during pregnancy and the postpartum period. *Journal of Obstetric, Gynecologic and Neonatal Nursing, 28,* 183–191.

McVeigh, C. (1997a). An Australian study of functional status after childbirth. *Midwifery, 13,* 172–178.

McVeigh, C. (1997b). Functional status after childbirth: A comparison of Australian women from English and non-English speaking backgrounds. *Australian College of Midwives Incorporated Journal, 10*(2), 15–21.

McVeigh, C. (1998). Functional status after childbirth in an Australian sample. *Journal of Obstetric, Gynecologic, and Neonatal Nursing, 27,* 402–409.

Mercer, R. T. (1986). *First-time motherhood.* New York: Springer Publishing.

Mercer, R. T. (1995). *Becoming a mother: Research on maternal identity from Rubin to the present.* New York: Springer Publishing.

Pugh, L. C., Milligan, R., Parks, P. L., Lenz, E. R., & Kitzman, H. (1999). Clinical approaches in the assessment of childbearing fatigue. *Journal of Obstetric, Gynecologic, and Neonatal Nursing, 28,* 74–80.

Reeder, S. J., Martin, L. L., & Koniak-Griffin, D. (1997). *Maternity nursing: Family, newborn, and women's health care* (18th ed.). Philadelphia: Lippincott-Raven.

Rubin, R. (1984). *Maternal identity and the maternal experience.* New York: Springer Publishing.

Ruchala, P. L., & Halstead, L. (1994). The postpartum experience of low-risk women: A time of adjustment and change. *Maternal-Child Nursing Journal, 22,* 83–89.

Sampselle, C. M., Seng, J., Yeo, S., Killion, C., & Oakley, D. (1999). Physical activity and postpartum well-being. *Journal of Obstetric, Gynecologic, and Neonatal Nursing, 28,* 41–49.

Smith-Hanrahan, C., & Deblois, D. (1995). Postpartum early discharge: Impact on maternal fatigue and functional ability. *Clinical Nursing Research, 4,* 50–66.

Troy, N. W., & Dalgas-Pelish, P. (1997). The natural evolution of postpartum fatigue among a group of primiparous women. *Clinical Nursing Research, 6,* 126–141.

Tulman, L., & Fawcett, J. (1988). Return of functional ability after childbirth. *Nursing Research, 37,* 77–81.

Tulman, L., Fawcett, J., Groblewski, L., & Silverman, L. (1990). Changes in functional status after childbirth. *Nursing Research, 39,* 70–75.

6

Changes in Women's Weight
After Delivery

Body weight is an important aspect of a woman's adaptation following childbirth. Yet, although some attention has been given to the pattern of weight loss—or gain—after childbirth, very little information is available about how a woman's body weight affects her adaptation during the postpartum.

In this chapter, we focus on changes in women's weight during the first six postpartum months, as well as on the relation of postpartum weight to physical health and functional status. In our Theory of Adaptation During Childbearing, we view postpartum weight as a focal stimulus that affects the adaptation responses of physical symptoms, physical energy, and functional status (Figures 6.1 and 6.2). As noted in chapter 3, our view of body weight as a focal stimulus is consistent with Roy's (1984) contention that one adaptation response can be viewed as a stimulus for another response. In keeping with the Roy Adaptation Model and the available evidence from the literature, we proposed that absolute weight, weight retained, and BMI weight classification at three and six weeks and three and six months postpartum, as well as weight lost at six weeks and three and six months postpartum would be related to functional status, physical symptoms, and physical energy (Figure 6.2).

POSTPARTUM WEIGHT CHANGES

Women generally expect to lose most, if not all, of the weight they gained during pregnancy in the months following childbirth. Women typically do lose between 19 and 24 pounds within the first few weeks after delivery—12 to 13 pounds are accounted for by the fetus, placenta, amniotic fluid, and delivery blood loss; 5 to 8 pounds by water loss through perspiration and diuresis during the first week of the postpartum, and 2 to 3 pounds by uterine involution and lochia (Reeder, Martin, & Koniak-Griffin, 1997).

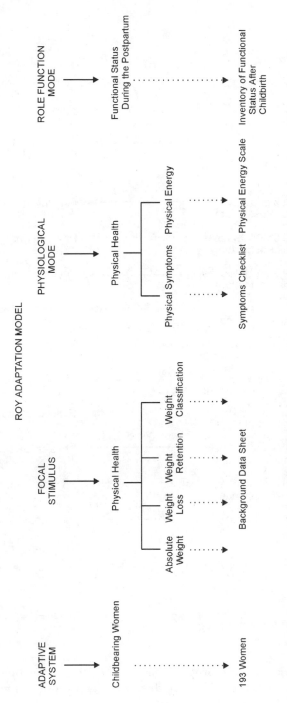

FIGURE 6.1 Linkages between the Roy Adaptation Model, physical health and functional status, and study variables and measures: Examination of the influence of postpartum body weight.

Roy Adaptation Model:

Changes in Stimuli ——————————————▶ Changes in Responses

Theory of Adaptation During Childbearing:

Weight ——————————————▶ Functional Status
Physical Health

Study Variables:

Absolute Weight at 3 and 6 Weeks ——————▶ Functional Status
and 3 and 6 Months Postpartum

Absolute Weight at 3 and 6 Weeks ——————▶ Physical Energy
and 3 and 6 Months Postpartum

Absolute Weight at 3 and 6 Weeks ——————▶ Physical Symptoms
and 3 and 6 Months Postpartum

Weight Lost at 6 Weeks and ——————————▶ Functional Status
3 Months and 6 Months Postpartum

Weight Lost at 6 Weeks and ——————————▶ Physical Energy
3 Months and 6 Months Postpartum

Weight Lost at 6 Weeks and ——————————▶ Physical Symptoms
3 Months and 6 Months Postpartum

Weight Retained at 3 and 6 Weeks —————▶ Functional Status
and 3 and 6 Months Postpartum

Weight Retained at 3 and 6 Weeks —————▶ Physical Energy
and 3 and 6 Months Postpartum

Weight Retained at 3 and 6 Weeks —————▶ Physical Symptoms
and 3 and 6 Months Postpartum

Postpartum Weight Classification at ————▶ Functional Status
3 and 6 Weeks and 3 and 6 Months
Postpartum

Postpartum Weight Classification at ————▶ Physical Energy
3 and 6 Weeks and 3 and 6 Months
Postpartum

Postpartum Weight Classification at ————▶ Physical Symptoms
3 and 6 Weeks and 3 and 6 Months
Postpartum

FIGURE 6.2 Diagrams of propositions of the Roy Adaptation Model, Theory of Adaptation During Childbearing, and postpartum weight variables.

Some women—especially those who gain more than the recommended amount during pregnancy (see chapter 3)—do not return to their prepregnancy weight (Brewer, Bates, & Vennoy, 1989; Parham, Astrom, & King, 1990). Experts estimate that, on average, women retain 2.2 pounds over their prepregnancy weight (Institute of Medicine, 1990), although researchers have found this to vary. Thorsdottir and Birgisdottir (1998) reported that the vast majority (88%) of 200 Icelandic women in their study returned to their prepregnancy weight within 18 to 24 months after delivery. Almost one-third (30%) of the 1,423 women in Ohlin and Rossner's (1990, 1994) study lost weight during the first year after childbirth. And, although two (4%) of the 56 women who participated in Brewer and colleagues' (1989) study gained weight during the first six postpartum months, and one woman had no change in her weight, the remainder lost from 4 to 46 pounds.

Retained weight generally is lost at a decelerating rate during the first year following childbirth (Brewer, Bates, & Vannoy, 1989; Walker, 1995). Sampselle and colleagues (1999) found that 1,003 women residing in the United States (U.S.) retained an average of 10.49 pounds over their prepregnancy weight at six weeks after delivery. To and Cheung (1998) reported that 292 Chinese women retained an average of eight pounds at three months postpartum. Schauberger, Rooney, and Brimer (1992) found that the 795 U.S. women they studied retained an average of three pounds from the first prenatal visit to six months postpartum. Ohlin and Rossner (1990) reported that their sample of 1,423 Swedish women had an average weight gain of 3.3 pounds over their prepregnancy weight one year after delivery. Another study of 149 U.S. women revealed an average weight gain of 5.5 pounds (range = −15 to 65 pounds) at one year postpartum (Walker, 1997). Findings from still another study of U.S. women, who were interviewed 10 to 18 months after childbirth, indicated that 56% of 1,599 White women retained fewer than four pounds over their prepregnancy weight, compared with 37% of 1,345 Black women. In addition, 25% of White women and 45% of Black women retained nine or more pounds (Keppel & Taffel, 1993).

Postpartum Weight and Method of Infant Feeding

Infant feeding is a potentially confounding variable in studies of postpartum weight. Studies designed to compare postpartum weight in women who breastfed and those who bottle fed their infants have, however, yielded conflicting findings. Brewer, Bates, and Vannoy (1989) reported that among a group of 56 women, the 21 women who breastfed exclusively for the first six months following delivery lost more weight ($M =$ 18.26 pounds) than the 15 women who bottle fed exclusively ($M = 18.02$ pounds) or the 20 women who initially breastfed and then bottle fed ($M = 15.88$ pounds). Similarly, Dewey, Heinig, and Nommsen (1993) found that the 46 women who breastfed their infants for at least six months lost more weight during the first postpartum year ($M = 9.68$ pounds) than the 39 women who bottle fed their infants ($M = 5.28$ pounds), primarily due to the weight lost during the third to sixth postpartum months. More specifically, at six months postpartum, breast feeding mothers weighed an average of 6.16 pounds less than their bottle feeding counterparts. In contrast, Chou, Chan, and Moyer-Mileur (1999) reported that at 12 weeks postpartum, a group of six women who bottle fed their infants had lost more weight than a group of 14 breastfeeding women ($p < .03$).

Postpartum Weight and Functional Status

No studies designed to directly examine the relation between postpartum weight and functional status were located. Some investigators have, however, examined the relation between postpartum weight and physical activity. The findings of those studies are conflicting. A few investigators have found a negative association between postpartum weight retention and physical activity. Sampselle and colleagues (1999) reported that more active women retained less weight at six weeks postpartum than their less active counterparts (8.6 pounds versus 11.3 pounds). Ohlin and Rossner (1994) reported that Swedish women who retained 11 pounds or more by the end of the first postpartum year were less physically active than women who retained less weight. Similarly, Walker and Freeland-Graves (1998) reported that bottle-feeding women with higher postpartum weight gains exercised less during the first four postpartum months than their bottle-feeding counterparts who did not retain weight and women who breastfed their infants. In contrast, other investigators have found no evidence of an association between postpartum weight classification and physical activity (Morin, Gennaro, & Fehder, 1999; Schauberger, Rooney, & Brimer, 1992).

Postpartum Weight, Physical Symptoms, and Physical Energy

No studies of the relation of postpartum weight to physical symptoms or physical energy could be located. Thus, our study results shed light on these important aspects of postpartum adaptation.

THE RESULTS OF OUR STUDY

Complete data for postpartum weight were available for 193 of the women in our study. We examined postpartum weight in four ways: absolute weight in pounds at three and six weeks and three and six months postpartum; number of pounds lost from three to six weeks, six weeks to three months, and three months to six months postpartum; number of pounds retained over prepregnancy weight at three and six weeks and three and six months postpartum; and Body Mass Index (BMI) classifications for underweight, normal weight, and overweight at three and six weeks and three and six months postpartum [BMI calculations are given in chapter 3].

Postpartum Weight and Infant Feeding

We initially examined the influence of infant feeding method on postpartum weight. The percentage of women who used each infant feeding method during the postpartum is given in Table 6.1. There were no statistically significant differences in absolute postpartum weight, weight loss, weight retention, or BMI classification among women who breastfed, bottle fed, or breast and bottle fed their infants at any time during the postpartum ($p > .05$). Therefore, our subsequent analyses included all of the women, regardless of infant feeding method.

TABLE 6.1 Infant Feeding Methods During the Postpartum ($N = 193$)

Feeding Method [%]	3 Weeks Postpartum	6 Weeks Postpartum	3 Months Postpartum	6 Months Postpartum
Breast	73.6%	61.7%	52.8%	43.5%
Bottle	14.0%	17.1%	24.4%	33.2%
Breast and Bottle	12.4%	21.2%	22.8%	23.3%

Changes in Postpartum Weight

The women's absolute weight ranged from 93 to 230 pounds at six months postpartum (Table 6.2). Their weight decreased progressively throughout the postpartum ($p < .0005$), with statistically significant decreases in absolute weight from three weeks to six weeks, six weeks to three months, and three months to six months.

Amount of weight lost or gained also changed during the postpartum ($p = .009$) (Table 6.2). On average, the women had lost slightly more than 1.5 pounds between three weeks and six weeks, slightly more than 2.5 pounds between six weeks and three months, and three pounds between three and six months postpartum. The only statistically significant difference was between six weeks and three months postpartum.

The amount of weight the women retained over their prepregnancy weight decreased steadily ($p < .0005$), with statistically significant decreases throughout the postpartum (Table 6.2). By six months after delivery, the women's weight ranged from 20 pounds less to 45 pounds more than their prepregnancy weight, with an average gain of five pounds.

We also calculated each woman's BMI to determine the percentage of women who were underweight, of normal weight, and overweight throughout the postpartum. Few women were classified as underweight (BMI < 19.8) at any time during the first six postpartum months—6% at three and six weeks, 8% at three months, and 15% at six months. More women were classified as overweight (BMI > 26.0)—29% at three weeks, 28% at six weeks, 24% at three months, and 19% at six months. The majority of women were classified as normal weight (BMI 19.8–26.0)—65% at three weeks, 66% at six weeks and six months, and 67% at three months.

Postpartum Weight and Functional Status

We looked at the correlations between absolute postpartum weight and functional status, postpartum weight loss and functional status, and postpartum weight retention and functional status during the postpartum (Table 6.3) [Our data for postpartum functional status are presented in chapter 5 (Table 5.1)]. All of the correlations were of very low magnitude. The only statistically significant correlation was for weight retention and functional status at three weeks postpartum

TABLE 6.2 Changes in Weight and Weight Retention During the Postpartum ($N = 193$)

Variable	3 Weeks Postpartum	6 Weeks Postpartum	3 Months Postpartum	6 Months Postpartum	p
Weight in pounds [M, SD, Range]	149.33 (25.72) 96 to 225	147.68 (25.60) 94 to 220	144.96 (25.44) 94 to 225	141.91 (25.48) 93 to 230	< .0005[a]
Weight loss/gain in pounds between intervals [M, SD, Range]	—	−1.65 (4.40) −18 to +20	−2.72 (4.50) −10 to +24	−3.05 (5.21) −10 to +20	.009[b]
Weight retention in pounds over prepregnancy weight [M, SD, Range]	12.51 (10.23) −15 to +46	+10.87 (10.11) −20 to +46	+8.16 (9.49) −19 to +46	+5.10 (9.18) −20 to +46	< .0005[a]

[a]Differences between 3 weeks and 6 weeks, 6 weeks and 3 months, and 3 months and 6 months statistically significant.
[b]Difference between 6 weeks and 3 months statistically significant.

TABLE 6.3   Correlations of Weight, Weight Loss, and Weight Retention with Functional Status, Physical Symptoms, and Physical Energy During the Postpartum ($N = 193$)

Variable	3 Weeks Postpartum Functional Status	6 Weeks Postpartum Functional Status	3 Months Postpartum Functional Status	6 Months Postpartum Functional Status
Weight	.042	.074	.059	.076
Weight Loss	—	−.053	−.046	.020
Weight Retention	−.177*	−.076	−.050	−.053
	Physical Symptoms	Physical Symptoms	Physical Symptoms	Physical Symptoms
Weight	.081	−.017	.022	.113
Weight Loss	—	.001	−.069	−.003
Weight Retention	.189**	−.048	.000	.108
	Physical Energy	Physical Energy	Physical Energy	Physical Energy
Weight	−.047	.054	.069	−.070
Weight Loss	—	.061	.087	.067
Weight Retention	−.109	−.068	.060	−.146*

*$p < .05$
**$p < .01$

($p < .05$), such that the fewer the pounds retained, the greater the level of performance of usual activities. Furthermore, there were no differences in level of functional status among the BMI classifications of underweight, normal weight, and overweight groups of women at any time during the postpartum.

However, when at six months postpartum, we asked the women what was hindering their return to their usual physical condition, slightly more that one fifth (21%) mentioned their weight. Typical comments were:

> "I am not at [my optimal] weight yet."
> "I haven't lost all the weight; it is going slowly."
> "I need to lose weight."

Some of the women cited a specific number of pounds they wanted to lose before they would feel that they had returned to their usual physical condition. One stated, "5 pounds to go." Elaborating, another women explained:

> I have 12 pounds to lose. I knew I would have to be patient with my weight and I would not be able to whip it off. . . . But then every once in a while I would look in the mirror and get so frustrated. That really upset me. Being a dancer, it was a very deep concern of mine, [and] it is a whole national health thing right now. I have been on a diet since 7th grade, so being heavy is a very big thing to me. I still have a whole wardrobe I haven't looked at in over a year because I can't get back into my clothes. I don't want to spend a lot of money on new clothes because when I get back to my weight I won't wear them. . . . I accepted the fact that it will take me a year to get back there. However, there are days when I don't want to accept that.

One woman's comments reflected a direct link between her current weight and performance of her usual personal care activities (exercise and diet). She explained, "In the beginning I did a lot of exercising when I could, and I think that helped me lose the weight right away. And . . . I was used to not eating a lot of food because of the diet [during pregnancy], and . . . so I lost my weight right away."

A few (2%) women noted that their current weight was one of the things that they liked less about life since delivery. One woman stated that although she had "lost most of the baby weight," she was "a little heavier than I was; there are a few pounds that I have to lose." Two women linked their appearance, which they liked less about life since delivery, with their weight. One commented that her current weight contributed negatively to her appearance. She stated, "I don't look as cute; I have gained a little more weight." The other woman attributed her appearance to the weight she had gained during pregnancy. She explained, "I feel I am less attractive because I still have the side effects of pregnancy—flab and stretch marks."

Although our quantitative data revealed no differences in postpartum weight for different infant feeding methods, two women linked their extra weight to breastfeeding. One commented, "Nursing . . . made me gain 20 pounds. Carrying around that extra weight was very depressing and debilitating." The other woman explained, "I am frustrated because I am overweight. But I can't do a lot with that until I am done nursing."

Postpartum Weight, Physical Symptoms, and Physical Energy

We also looked at the correlations between postpartum weight and physical symptoms and physical energy (Table 6.3) [Our data for postpartum physical symptoms and physical energy are presented in chapter 5 (Table 5.1)]. All of the correlations were low in magnitude. One statistically significant correlation indicated an association between a higher number of pounds retained and an increased number of physical symptoms at three weeks postpartum ($p < .01$). The only other statistically significant correlation indicated an association between a higher number of pounds retained and a lower the level of physical energy at six months postpartum ($p < .05$).

In addition, we explored the association between BMI classification and physical symptoms and physical energy. There were no differences in the number of physical symptoms or the levels of physical energy among the underweight, normal weight, and overweight groups of women at any time during the postpartum.

When interviewed at six months postpartum, one woman's comment reflected a link between her weight and tiredness, which can be considered a proxy for physical energy. She stated, "I am trying to lose weight and I still feel tired."

CONCLUSION

The results for this part of our study lend little support to the credibility of the Roy Adaptation Model proposition asserting that one adaptation response can be a focal stimulus that influences other adaptation responses. More specifically, the results do not support the part of our Theory of Adaptation During Childbearing addressing the influence of physical health, in the form of body weight variables, on other physical health variables (physical symptoms and physical energy) and functional status. Instead, our findings revealed that the focal stimulus of postpartum weight had minimal influence on the role function mode response of functional status and the physiological mode responses of physical symptoms and physical energy. Weight retention was the only body weight variable that was correlated with functional status, physical symptoms, and physical energy, and there was no consistent pattern of statistically significant correlations throughout the postpartum (Table 6.3). Furthermore, the correlations were so low that they are clinically meaningless.

Approximately two thirds of the women in our study were of normal weight according to BMI classification throughout the first six postpartum months. A similar percentage of the women were in the same BMI classification for their prepregnancy weight (see chapter 3). These data indicate that there may have been insufficient variability in our sample to adequately test the influence of body weight on adaptation responses. Future studies, therefore, should be designed to purposively sample larger numbers of women who are underweight, overweight, and obese.

Our data do not support previous findings of an association between infant feeding method and postpartum weight. Although previous studies have revealed that women who breastfeed their infants retained more weight or less weight than women who bottle fed, our findings yielded no associations between method of infant feeding and absolute postpartum weight, weight loss, weight retention, or BMI classification at any time during the first six postpartum months. Noteworthy is the fact that our study sample of 193 women was considerably larger than the samples for previous studies (Brewer, Bates, & Vannoy, 1989 [$N = 36$]; Dewey, Heinig, & Nommsen, 1993 [$N = 85$]; Chou, Chan, & Moyer-Mileur, 1999 [$N = 20$]).

Our findings revealed that, on average, the women who participated in our study experienced a progressive loss of weight throughout the first six postpartum months. Yet even by six months postpartum, the women retained an average of 5.10 pounds (Table 6.2) over their prepregnancy weight. Our data for weight retention at six weeks (10.87 pounds) and three months (8.16 pounds) are remarkably similar to Sampselle and colleagues' (1999) finding of 10.49 pounds retained at six weeks and To and Cheung's (1998) finding of 8 pounds retained at three months.

Researchers should consider conducting long-term longitudinal studies to track changes in women's weight after the birth of each child. Researchers also should consider comparing weight changes in women who have given birth with those who have not. Indeed, research already has revealed that during their adult lives, women who have given birth gain, on average, more weight than women who have not had children. Women frequently experience a persistent weight increase over prepregnancy weight and a redistribution of adipose tissue after their first pregnancy (Smith et al., 1994). Furthermore, the findings of a longitudinal study (Williamson et al., 1994) revealed that among a group of 2,547 White women aged 25 to 45 years, those who did not give birth during the 10-year study period gained less weight ($M = 3.5$ pounds) than those had given birth during that time ($M = 4.1$ pounds). In addition, the women who had given birth to three children during the study period gained more weight ($M = 4.84$ pounds) than those who had given birth to one or two children ($M = 3.74$).

More needs to be known about the extent to which women are satisfied with their weight following childbirth. In a ground-breaking study of 227 women, Walker (1998) found that almost one quarter (22%) of the women reported that they were satisfied with their postpartum weight but wanted to lose more weight; two fifths (40%) were overweight with mild dissatisfaction, and almost one tenth (8%) reported weight-related distress. There was, however, a substantial overlap across the women's BMI classification group and their reports of satisfaction, dissatisfaction, and distress. Although we did not measure the women's satisfaction with their postpartum weight, during the six months postpartum interview some women told us that their weight was one of the things that they liked less about their life after childbirth, which reflects their dissatisfaction with their weight. Researchers should, therefore, follow Walker's lead and include a measure of satisfaction with weight in their studies of postpartum weight changes.

REFERENCES

Brewer, M. M., Bates, M. R., & Vannoy, L. P. (1989). Postpartum changes in maternal weight and body fat deposits in lactating versus non-lactating women. *American Journal of Clinical Nutrition, 49,* 259–265.

Chou, T. W., Chan, G. M., & Moyer-Mileur, L. (1999). Postpartum body composition changes in lactating and non-lactating primiparas. *Nutrition, 15,* 481–484.

Dewey, K. G., Heinig, M. J., & Nommsen, L. A. (1993). Maternal weight-loss patterns during prolonged lactation. *American Journal of Clinical Nutrition, 58,* 162–166.

Institute of Medicine. (1990). *Nutrition during pregnancy: Weight gain and nutrients.* Washington, DC: National Academy Press.

Keppel, K. G., & Taffel, S. M. (1993). Pregnancy-related weight gain and retention: Implications of the 1990 Institute of Medicine guidelines. *American Journal of Public Health, 83,* 1100–1103.

Morin, K., Gennaro, S., & Fehder, W. (1999). Nutrition and exercise in overweight and obese postpartum women. *Applied Nursing Research, 12,* 13–21.

Ohlin, A., & Rossner, S. (1990). Maternal body weight development after pregnancy. *International Journal of Obesity, 14,* 159–173.

Ohlin, A., & Rossner, S. (1994). Trends in eating patterns, physical activity and sociodemographic factors in relation to postpartum body weight development. *British Journal of Nutrition, 71,* 457–470.

Parham, E. S., Astrom, M. F., & King, S. H. (1990). The association of pregnancy weight gain with the mother's postpartum weight. *Journal of the American Dietetic Association, 90,* 550–554.

Reeder, S. J., Martin, L. L., & Koniak-Griffin, D. (1997). *Maternity nursing: Family, newborn, and women's health care* (18th ed.). Philadelphia: Lippincott-Raven.

Roy, C. (1984). *Introduction to nursing: An adaptation model* (2nd ed.). Englewood Cliffs, NJ: Prentice-Hall.

Sampselle, C. M., Seng, J., Yeo, S., Killion, C., & Oakley, D. (1999). Physical activity and postpartum well-being. *Journal of Obstetric, Gynecologic, and Neonatal Nursing, 28,* 41–49.

Schauberger, C. W., Rooney, B. L., & Brimer, L. M. (1992). Factors that influence weight loss in the puerperium. *Obstetrics and Gynecology, 79,* 424–429.

Smith, D. E., Lewis, C. E., Caveny, J. L., Perkins, L. L., Burke, G. L., & Bild, D. E. (1994). Longitudinal changes in adiposity associated with pregnancy: The CARDIA study—Coronary Artery Risk Development in Young Adults Study. *Journal of the American Medical Association, 271,* 1747–1751.

Thorsdottir, I., & Birgisdottir, B. E. (1998). Different weight gain in women of normal weight before pregnancy: Postpartum weight and birth weight. *Obstetrics and Gynecology, 92,* 377–383.

To, W. W., & Cheung, W. (1998). The relationship between weight gain in pregnancy, birth weight, and postpartum weight retention. *Australian and New Zealand Journal of Obstetrics and Gynaecology, 38,* 176–179.

Walker, L. O. (1995). Weight gain after childbirth: A women's health concern? *Annals of Behavioral Medicine, 17,* 132–141.

Walker, L. O. (1997). Weight and weight-related distress after childbirth: Relationships to stress, social support, and depressive symptoms. *Journal of Holistic Nursing, 15,* 389–405.

Walker, L. O. (1998). Weight-related distress in the early months after childbirth. *Western Journal of Nursing Research, 20,* 30–44.

Walker, L. O., & Freeland-Graves, J. (1998). Lifestyle factors related to postpartum weight gain and body image in bottle- and breastfeeding women. *Journal of Obstetric, Gynecologic, and Neonatal Nursing, 27,* 151–160.

Williamson, D. F., Madans, J., Pamuk, E., Flegal, K. M., Kendrick, J. S., & Serdula, M. K. (1994). A prospective study of childbearing and 10-year weight gain in U.S. white women 25 to 45 years of age. *International Journal of Obesity and Related Metabolic Disorders, 18,*561–569.

7

Feelings about Motherhood, Family Relationships, and Functional Status

The postpartum is a prolonged period of change for a woman and her family. Indeed, "The postpartum period is neither short nor static; rather, it is a period characterized by dynamic changes in the women's mental and physical health that may persist for months" (Gjerdingen, Froberg, & Fontaine, 1990, p. 82).

Changes in physical health during the postpartum were discussed in chapters 5 and 6. In this chapter, we present the part of our Theory of Adaptation During Childbearing dealing with psychosocial health, family relationships, and their relation to functional status during the first six months of the postpartum (Figures 7.1 and 7.2). In keeping with the Roy Adaptation Model and the available evidence from the literature, we proposed that several psychosocial health variables, including psychological symptoms (feeling anxious, feeling depressed, feeling better than usual), gratification with labor and delivery, life satisfaction, satisfaction with motherhood, and maternal confidence in ability to cope with tasks of motherhood would change during the postpartum (Figure 7.2 [A]). We also proposed that five family relationships variables—support from family and friends, quality of the marital relationship after delivery, maternal perception of father's participation in child care, maternal perception of infant temperament, and maternal reports of infant nocturnal sleep—would change during the postpartum (Figure 7.2 [A]). Furthermore, we proposed that all of those psychosocial health variables and family relationships variables would be related to functional status at three weeks, six weeks, three months, and six months postpartum (Figure 7.2 [B, C]).

PSYCHOSOCIAL HEALTH DURING THE POSTPARTUM

The postpartum is a time of considerable psychological and social change, as the woman and her family adjust to the new member. Thus,

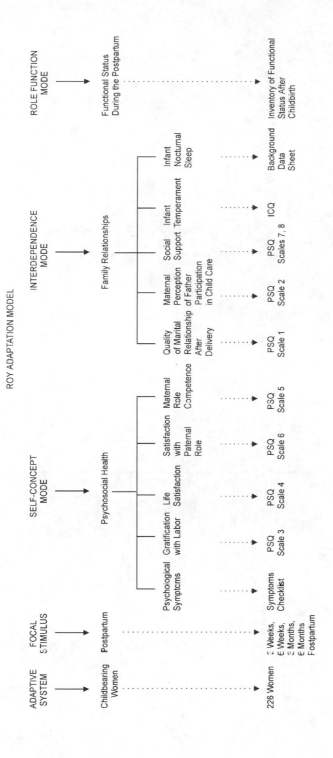

FIGURE 7.1   Linkages between the Roy Adaptation Model, psychosocial health, family relationships, and functional status, and study variables and measures.

Legend:
PSQ = Postpartum Self-Evaluation Questionnaire
ICQ = Infant Characteristics Questionnaire

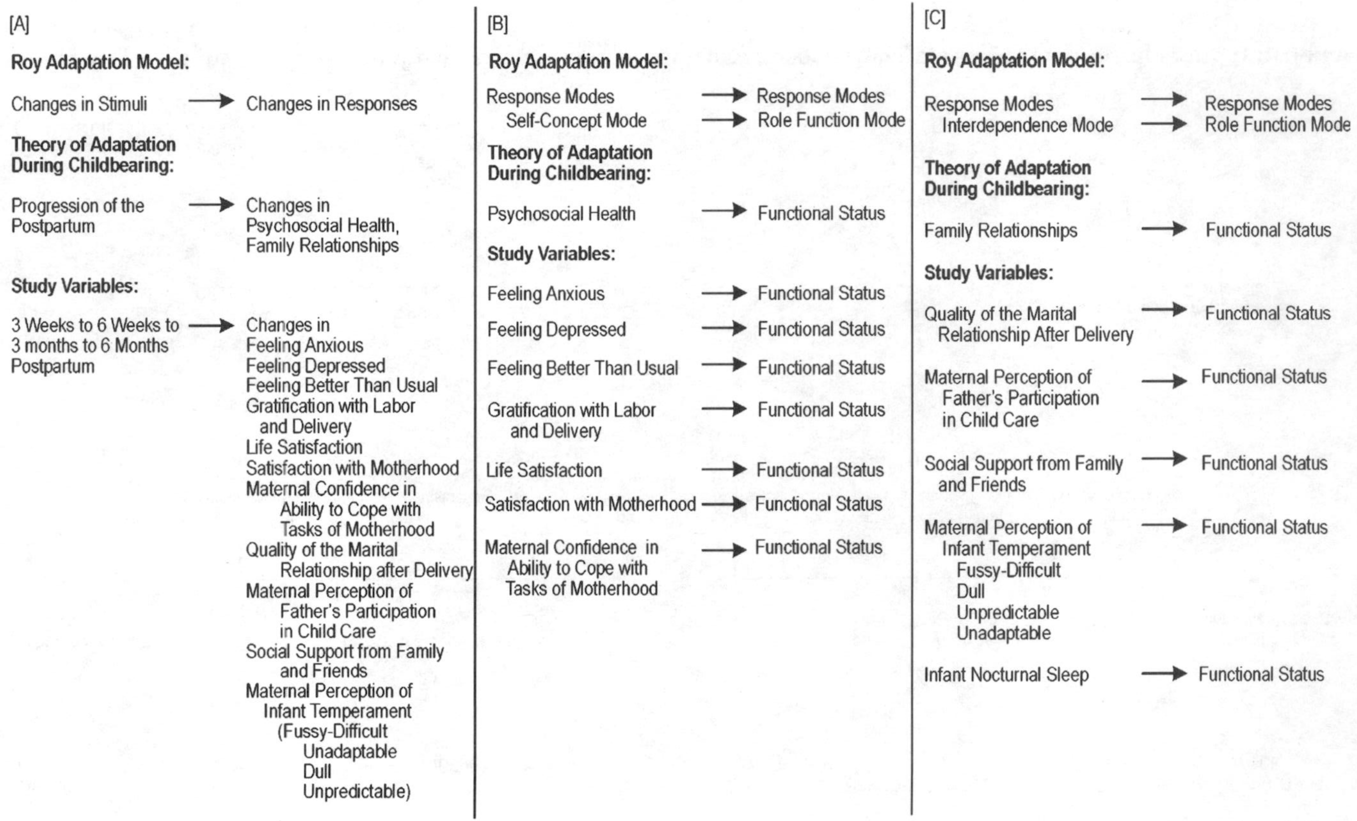

[A]

Roy Adaptation Model:

Changes in Stimuli → Changes in Responses

Theory of Adaptation During Childbearing:

Progression of the Postpartum → Changes in Psychosocial Health, Family Relationships

Study Variables:

3 Weeks to 6 Weeks to 3 months to 6 Months Postpartum → Changes in Feeling Anxious Feeling Depressed Feeling Better Than Usual Gratification with Labor and Delivery Life Satisfaction Satisfaction with Motherhood Maternal Confidence in Ability to Cope with Tasks of Motherhood Quality of the Marital Relationship after Delivery Maternal Perception of Father's Participation in Child Care Social Support from Family and Friends Maternal Perception of Infant Temperament (Fussy-Difficult Unadaptable Dull Unpredictable)

[B]

Roy Adaptation Model:

Response Modes Self-Concept Mode → Response Modes Role Function Mode

Theory of Adaptation During Childbearing:

Psychosocial Health → Functional Status

Study Variables:

Feeling Anxious → Functional Status

Feeling Depressed → Functional Status

Feeling Better Than Usual → Functional Status

Gratification with Labor and Delivery → Functional Status

Life Satisfaction → Functional Status

Satisfaction with Motherhood → Functional Status

Maternal Confidence in Ability to Cope with Tasks of Motherhood → Functional Status

[C]

Roy Adaptation Model:

Response Modes Interdependence Mode → Response Modes Role Function Mode

Theory of Adaptation During Childbearing:

Family Relationships → Functional Status

Study Variables:

Quality of the Marital Relationship After Delivery → Functional Status

Maternal Perception of Father's Participation in Child Care → Functional Status

Social Support from Family and Friends → Functional Status

Maternal Perception of Infant Temperament Fussy-Difficult Dull Unpredictable Unadaptable → Functional Status

Infant Nocturnal Sleep → Functional Status

FIGURE 7.2 Diagrams of propositions of the Roy Adaptation Model, the Theory of Adaptation During Childbearing, and study variables: Functional status, psychosocial health, and family relationships during the postpartum.

our study included several variables that reflect postpartum psychosocial health.

Psychological Symptoms

We continued our interest in the three psychological symptoms that we examined during pregnancy (chapter 4)—anxiety, depression, and feeling better than usual. Anxiety is frequently reported during the postpartum, although at low levels. Fawcett and York (1986) found that almost two thirds (61%) of 23 women who participated in their study experienced anxiety at some time during the first six postpartum weeks. Although there is some evidence that the level of anxiety declines gradually as the postpartum progresses (Gjerdingen & Chaloner, 1994b; Singh & Sexena, 1991), Gennaro (1988) reported continued low levels of anxiety from the first through the seventh week after delivery.

Depression is a relatively frequently reported psychological symptom of the postpartum, although the level of depression typically is low to moderate (Gennaro, 1988; Hughes, Turton, & Evans, 1999; Parisher, Nasrallah, & Gardner, 1997; Ruchala & Halstead, 1994). The level of depression, however, tends to vary throughout the postpartum. Gjerdingen, Froberg, and Kochevar (1991) found that, on average, depressive symptoms peaked at the sixth postpartum week and then declined steadily at three and six months postpartum. Affonso and colleagues (1993) found considerable variation in the number and type of depressive symptoms when measured at one to two weeks and 14 weeks following delivery. In contrast, Koenigseder (1991) found no evidence of any weekly change in consistently low levels of depression throughout the first six postpartum weeks.

The number and type of postpartum depressive symptoms have led to classifications ranging from "baby blues" to postpartum psychosis (Beck, Reynolds, & Rutowski, 1992; Reeder, Martin, & Koniak-Griffin, 1997; Wolman, Chalmers, Hofmeyr, & Nikodem, 1993). The "baby blues" or "maternity blues" generally are transient, typically occur within the first ten days following delivery, and last approximately one to ten days (Beck, 1991; Pitt, 1973; Reeder, Martin, & Koniak-Griffin, 1997). Reports of the rate of maternity blues experienced by women following delivery range from a low of 15% to a high of 66% (Harris et al., 1994; Murata, Nadaoka, Morioka, Oiji, & Saito, 1998). In contrast, postpartum psychosis is very rare, occurring in just 0.1% to 0.2% of women (Beck, 1999).

Postpartum depression, which is classified as a nonpsychotic postpartum mood disorder (Beck, 1999), is experienced by anywhere from 3% to 27% of women (Bryan et al., 1999); the average rate has been calculated at 13% (O'Hara & Swain, 1996). This type of depression typically begins within four weeks of delivery, is relatively mild, and may persist for many months (Beck, 1999; Koenigseder, 1991; Reeder, Martin, & Koniak-Griffin, 1997; Whiffen & Gotlib, 1993). There is some evidence of a link between maternity blues and postpartum depression. In particular, Beck, Reynolds, and Rutowski (1992) reported that women who experience more severe maternity blues are at increased risk for depression later in the postpartum.

Postpartum depression has been noted to occur but vary in intensity in women from various countries. The findings from a study of 892 women from nine countries that represented five continents revealed that women residing in European countries and Australia had the lowest levels of postpartum depression, whereas women residing in Asian and South American countries had the highest levels. Women residing in the United States reported moderate levels of postpartum depression (Affonso, De, Horowitz, & Mayberry, 2000).

Affonso, Lovett, Paul, and Sheptak (1990) pointed out that the physical symptoms experienced during the postpartum may mimic the symptoms of depression, leading to both overdiagnosis and underdiagnosis of clinical depression following delivery. It is imperative, then, that distinctions be made between physical and psychological symptoms after delivery.

Bergant, Heim, Ulmer, and Illmensee (1999) found that 20% of the 1,250 women in their study experienced what they labeled as early postnatal depressive mood on the fifth postpartum day. Fishbein and Burggraf (1998) found that 25% of the women in their study "said they were depressed or experiencing the 'baby blues' " two weeks after delivery (p. 145). Hughes, Turton, and Evans (1999) reported that although just 5% of the women in their study experienced a high level of depression at six weeks postpartum, the rate increased to 12% at six months postpartum. Both O'Hara (1986) and Allen (1999) reported that 12% of the women who participated in their studies experienced postpartum depression within the first two months following delivery. Gotlib, Wiffen, Mount, Milne, and Cordy (1989) found that approximately 25% of the 360 women who participated in their study experienced depressive symptomatology following delivery; however, just 7% of those women met the diagnostic criteria for depression. Gjerdingen and Chaloner (1994b) reported that the women in their study experienced a higher level of depression at one month postpartum than at six, nine, or twelve months.

More than two fifths (43%) of the 23 women in Fawcett and York's (1986) study reported feeling depressed during the first six weeks of the postpartum. Fawcett and York did not, however, further classify the women's feelings of depression as "baby blues," postpartum depression, or postpartum psychosis. Our study also did not utilize a classification system for the women's feelings of depression; however, we tracked the changes in the reports of feelings of depression from three weeks to six months postpartum.

Feeling better than usual is another psychological symptom experienced by some women during the postpartum (Drake, Verhulst, & Fawcett, 1988). Although we have not found any longitudinal studies of changes in feeling better than usual during the postpartum, we speculated that this psychological symptom would vary as the postpartum progressed.

Psychological Symptoms and Functional Status

Limited empirical evidence documents the influence of psychological symptoms on functional status during the postpartum. Gjerdingen and Chaloner (1994b) reported that women's overall mental health was related to their performance of recreational activities at one month after delivery. McVeigh (2000a) found statistically significant negative correlations between anxiety and functional status at six weeks, three months, and six months postpartum, such that greater maternal anxiety was related to a lower level of functional status. Noteworthy is McVeigh's use of the *Inventory of Functional Status After Childbirth* (IFSAC), the instrument we used to measure postpartum functional status.

The symptoms of depression overlap with the performance of usual activities of daily living included in our definition and measurement of functional status (see Appendix, Table A.1). Thus, it is reasonable to speculate that a higher level of depression would be associated with a lower level of functional status throughout the postpartum. Although Koenigseder (1991) found evidence of such a relation, it was statistically significant only on the third postpartum day and not at any other time during the first six postpartum weeks.

PSQ Psychosocial Health Variables

Our interest in postpartum psychosocial health extended beyond psychological symptoms to those that Lederman, Weingarten, and Lederman (1981) included in the *Postpartum Self-Evaluation Questionnaire* (PSQ)—gratification with labor and delivery, life satisfaction, satisfaction with motherhood, and maternal confidence in ability to cope with tasks of motherhood. The definition of each of those variables is given in the Appendix (Table A.1).

Our review of studies that employed the PSQ revealed that women typically report relatively positive evaluations of those aspects of psychosocial health at two weeks (Oshio, 1992), six weeks (Halman, Oakley, & Lederman, 1995; Sampselle, Seng, Yeo, Killion, & Oakley, 1999; Weiss, 1991), four months (Reece & Harkless, 1998), and eight to nine months postpartum (Darling-Fisher, 1987). Changes in some of the variables included in the PSQ have been documented. Lederman and Lederman (1987) reported greater maternal confidence in ability to cope with tasks of motherhood but less satisfaction with motherhood at six weeks postpartum when compared with three days after delivery. In our earlier study of postpartum women, we detected no overall change between three weeks and six months postpartum in gratification with the labor and delivery experience or in life satisfaction (Tulman, Fawcett, Groblewski, & Silverman, 1990). We did, however, find significant overall changes in both maternal confidence and satisfaction with motherhood. More specifically, confidence in motherhood increased from three to six weeks postpartum and from six weeks to three months postpartum; there was no significant change from three to six months postpartum. Satisfaction with motherhood increased from six weeks to three months postpartum.

Using a different instrument, Mercer and Ferketich (1994) found that maternal role competence, which is conceptually similar to the PSQ maternal confidence variable, decreased from the time of delivery to one month postpartum but then progressively increased at four and eight months postpartum. Using still another instrument, Gjerdingen and Chaloner (1994b) found no differences in women's life satisfaction at one, three, six, nine, and twelve months postpartum.

PSQ Psychosocial Health Variables and Functional Status

Very little empirical evidence of the influence of the PSQ psychosocial variables on postpartum functional status is available. Data from our earlier longitudinal study (Tulman, Fawcett, Groblewski, & Silverman, 1990) indicated that greater maternal confidence in ability to cope with tasks of motherhood was related to higher levels of functional status in the areas of household, social and community, and personal care activities at six weeks postpartum. At three months postpartum, greater maternal confidence was related to increased functional status in the areas of social and community and personal care activities. At six months postpartum, greater maternal confidence and a higher level of satisfaction with motherhood were related to higher levels of functional status in the areas of household, personal care, and infant care activities. In addition, a higher level of satisfaction with motherhood was related to a higher level of functional status in the area of social and community activities at six months after delivery. Sampselle and colleagues' (1999) data support the existence of a positive relation between PSQ scores for gratification with labor and delivery, life satisfaction, satisfaction with motherhood, and maternal confidence in ability to cope with tasks of motherhood, and physical activity, which could be considered a proxy for functional status.

FAMILY RELATIONSHIPS DURING THE POSTPARTUM

PSQ Family Relationships Variables

Our interest in family relationships encompassed those variables included in the PSQ—quality of the marital relationship after delivery, maternal perception of the father's participation in child care, and social support from family and friends. Empirical evidence documents changes in some of these variables. The 54 women who participated in Lederman and Lederman's (1987) study reported greater dissatisfaction with the marital relationship, husband participation in child care, and social support from family and friends, as measured by the PSQ, at six weeks postpartum when compared with three days after delivery. Mercer, Ferketich, and DeJoseph (1993) reported that the partner relationship was more positive during pregnancy and postpartum hospitalization than at four and eight months postpartum. In another study, Mercer and Ferketich (1995) found that social support decreased progressively from one to four to eight months postpartum.

McVeigh (2000b) found that women reported a statistically significant decrease in satisfaction with support from partner and from others during the first six postpartum months. Similarly, Gjerdingen and Chaloner's (1994a) study findings revealed statistically significant declines in how often husbands, friends, and relatives expressed caring and how often friends and relatives provided practical help during the first postpartum year.

In our earlier study, we found no changes throughout the first six postpartum months in the marital relationship or in maternal perception of the husband's participation in child care (Tulman, Fawcett, Groblewski, & Silverman, 1990). We did, however, find significant improvement in social support from family and friends between three weeks and six weeks postpartum, but no significant changes at three months or six months after delivery.

PSQ Family Relationships Variables and Functional Status

The findings of our earlier study, in which we also used the PSQ, revealed that maternal perception of a higher level of father's participation in child care was associated with increased functional status in the area of social and community activities at six months postpartum (Tulman, Fawcett, Groblewski, & Silverman, 1990). Sampselle and colleagues (1999) reported evidence of a positive relation between the PSQ score for maternal perception of the father's participation in child care and physical activity at six weeks postpartum.

The quality of the marital relationship also has been linked with postpartum functioning. The evidence from our earlier study indicated that a higher quality of a woman's relationship with her husband, as measured by the PSQ, was related to a higher level of functional status in the areas of personal care and social and community activities at three months postpartum (Tulman, Fawcett, Groblewski, & Silverman, 1990). Sampselle and colleagues (1999) found evidence of a positive relation between the PSQ scores for quality of the woman's relationship with her husband and physical activity at six weeks postpartum.

Mercer (1995) implied that social support is linked with functional status. Norbeck and Tilden's (1983) data indicated that social support was inversely related to maternal perinatal and neonatal complications, which, in turn, are thought to influence functional status. Using the PSQ and the IFSAC, we previously found that greater social support was associated with increased functional status in the areas of social and community and infant care activities at six months postpartum

(Tulman, Fawcett, Groblewski, & Silverman, 1990). In contrast, Sampselle and colleagues (1999) found no evidence of relation between the PSQ score for social support from family and friends and physical activity at six weeks after delivery.

McVeigh (2000b) found some evidence of a relation between satisfaction with social support and functional status, as measured by the IFSAC. In particular, her study findings indicated that greater satisfaction with partner support was associated with decreased performance of infant care activities at six weeks postpartum, increased performance of personal care activities at three months postpartum, and increased performance of social and community activities at six months postpartum. In contrast, there was no evidence of a relation between satisfaction with support from others and functional status. McVeigh (1997a, 1997b) also reported that women who lacked support during the postpartum had a lower level of functional status in the areas of social and community activities than their counterparts who had support.

Infant Temperament

We regard maternal perception of infant temperament as a family relationships variable. Temperament is a general term that refers to "the *how* of behavior . . . the *way* in which an individual behaves (Thomas, Chess, & Birch, 1968, p. 4). The focus, then, is on individual differences in behavioral style rather than the content of behavior (Bates, 1987; Carey, 1983; Hubert, Wachs, Peters-Martin, & Gandour, 1982). Most questionnaires and other approaches to the measurement of temperament reflect a multidimensional view of temperament as a behavioral style. Furthermore, several techniques permit dichotomization of temperament into easy and difficult categories. Although there is some disagreement regarding the number and content of the dimensions of temperament (Bates, 1987; Hubert, Wachs, Peters-Martin, & Gandour, 1982), most researchers agree that difficult temperament is characterized primarily by negative affect, such as fussiness and crying, as well as irregularity of biological functions, tendency to withdraw from new situations and stimuli, slow adaptability to change, and tendencies to intense expressiveness. Easy temperament, in contrast, is characterized by positive affect, regularity, approach responses, quick adaptability, mild or moderate expressiveness, and positive mood responses.

Temperament often is regarded as a consistent core of personality that, paradoxically, varies with development (Bates, 1987). Empirical evidence suggests that changes in temperament are common during the first year of the infant's life (Hubert & Wachs, 1985). More specifically, changes in the direction of less difficult temperament with the infant's advancing age have been reported (Koniak-Griffin & Ludington-Hoe, 1988; Vaughn, Deinard, & Egeland, 1980). In an earlier study, we found that mothers perceived their six-month-old infants as less difficult than they had been at three months, and less fussy, unpredictable, and placid at three months than they had been at six weeks (Gennaro, Tulman, & Fawcett, 1990).

Infant Temperament and Functional Status

Infant temperament has been found to affect parents' interaction with their newborn (Bates, Freeland, & Lounsbury, 1979; Thomas, Chess, & Korn, 1982). The data from our earlier study indicated that maternal perception of infant temperament, as measured by infant unpredictability, fussiness, and unadaptability, was related to the woman's functional status (Tulman, Fawcett, Groblewski, & Silverman, 1990). More specifically, infant unpredictability was found to be negatively associated with functioning in household, social and community, and personal care activities at six weeks postpartum and with social and community and personal activities at three months postpartum. At six months postpartum, infant fussiness, unpredictability, and unadaptability were negatively associated with the level of functional status in household, personal care, and infant care activities. Infant fussiness and unadaptability were negatively associated with the level of functional status in social and community and infant care activities at that time as well.

Infant Nocturnal Sleep Patterns

We regard infant nocturnal sleep patterns as another family relationships variable. Although infants typically sleep between 12 and 20 hours each day, they display considerable variation in their sleep and waking states (Martin & Reeder, 1991; Reeder, Martin, & Koniak-Griffin, 1997). Inasmuch as few infants sleep through the night for the first several weeks after birth, it is not surprising that anecdotal reports indicate that many parents regard the first full night of sleep by their baby as a cause for celebration. As part of our study, we examined the women's reports of infant nocturnal sleep during the first six postpartum months. In particular, we examined the time after birth when the infant starts to sleep through the night.

Infant Nocturnal Sleep Patterns and Functional Status

Little attention has been given to the effect of infant nocturnal sleep on the woman's functional status. The authors of one textbook pointed out that the newborn infant's erratic schedule and need for attention and food frequently lead to maternal sleep deprivation, which, in turn, leads to changes in mood and cognitive functioning (Reeder, Martin, & Koniak-Griffin, 1997). They did not, however, indicate whether the infant's sleep patterns influence performance of any of the woman's usual activities throughout the postpartum. Evidence from a few studies supports the contention that infant nocturnal sleep is associated with the woman's functional status. In an earlier study, we found that less infant nighttime waking was associated with a higher level of functional status in the areas of household, personal care, and infant care activities at six months after delivery (Tulman, Fawcett, Groblewski, & Silverman, 1990). McVeigh (1997a) reported that women whose infants slept four hours or less between feedings at night had a lower level of functional status in the areas of household and personal care activities than did their counterparts whose infants slept more than four hours. McVeigh (1997b) also found that fewer women whose infants slept four hours or less between feedings at night returned to work by six weeks postpartum than women whose infants slept more than four hours.

THE RESULTS OF OUR STUDY

We examined the data from the 226 women who remained in our study throughout the postpartum for changes in psychosocial health and family relationships (Tables 7.1 and 7.3). We also examined the correlations of variables reflecting psychosocial health and family relationships with functional status throughout the first six months of the postpartum (Tables 7.2 and 7.4). [See our data for functional status in chapter 5 (Table 5.1).] In addition, we analyzed the women's responses to an interview that we conducted six months after delivery. They told us how their psychosocial health and their family relationships helped them

TABLE 7.1   Changes in Psychosocial Health Variables and Family Relationship Variables During the Postpartum (N = 226)

Variable	3 Weeks Postpartum	6 Weeks Postpartum	3 Months Postpartum	6 Months Postpartum	p
Psychological Symptoms [%]					
Feeling Anxious	53%	35%	24%	18%	< .0005[a]
Feeling Depressed	25%	21%	18%	18%	.065
Feeling Better Than Usual	23%	26%	27%	18%	.053
Postpartum Self-Evaluation Questionnaire Psychosocial Health Variables [M, SD]					
Gratification with Labor and Delivery*****	15.26 (5.72)	14.80 (5.79)	14.46 (5.74)	14.34 (5.80)	< .0005[b]
Life Satisfaction*****	19.19 (5.58)	19.20 (5.89)	19.24 (5.95)	19.40 (6.06)	.785
Satisfaction with Motherhood**	18.68 (4.44)	18.57 (4.48)	18.04 (4.46)	18.18 (4.20)	.024[c]
Maternal Confidence in Ability to Cope with Tasks of Motherhood*	23.06 (5.78)	21.26 (5.33)	19.85 (5.08)	19.39 (4.61)	< .0005[a]
Postpartum Self-Evaluation Questionnaire Family Relationships Variables [M, SD]					
Quality of Marital Relationship After Delivery***	16.01 (4.63)	16.51 (4.87)	16.41 (5.33)	16.63 (5.55)	.106
Father Participation in Child Care****	14.70 (4.67)	15.31 (5.05)	14.99 (5.11)	15.02 (5.05)	.044[b]
Social Support from Family and Friends***	15.76 (4.02)	15.69 (4.45)	15.58 (4.55)	15.50 (4.25)	.631

[a]Differences between 3 weeks and 6 weeks, and 6 weeks and 3 months statistically significant.
[b]Difference between 3 weeks and 6 weeks statistically significant.
[c]Differences between 6 weeks and 3 months statistically significant.
*Potential range of scores = 14–56; lower scores indicate more positive evaluation.
**Potential range of scores = 13–52; lower scores indicate more positive evaluation.
***Potential range of scores = 12–48; lower scores indicate more positive evaluation.
****Potential range of scores = 11–44; lower scores indicate more positive evaluation.
*****Potential range of scores = 10–40; lower scores indicate more positive evaluation.

TABLE 7.2 Correlations of Psychosocial Health and Family Relationship Variables With Functional Status During the Postpartum ($N = 226$)

Variable	3 Weeks Postpartum Functional Status	6 Weeks Postpartum Functional Status	3 Months Postpartum Functional Status	6 Months Postpartum Functional Status
Psychological Symptoms				
Feeling Anxious	−.320***	−.160*	−.200**	−.300***
Feeling Depressed	−.203**	−.189***	−.188***	−.270***
Feeling Fetter Than Usual	.045	.023	−.074	−.027
Postpartum Self-Evaluation Questionnaire Psychosocial Health Variables				
Gratification with Labor and Delivery	−.128	−.083	−.123	−.069
Life Satisfaction	−.103	−.048	−.060	−.075
Satisfaction with Motherhood	−.213**	−.237***	−.168*	−.211**
Maternal Confidence in Ability to Cope with Tasks of Motherhood	−.171**	−.194**	−.142*	−.231***
Postpartum Self-Evaluation Questionnaire Family Relationships Variables				
Quality of Marital Relationship After Delivery	−.063	−.089	−.191**	−.042
Father Participation in Child Care	.093	−.057	−.084	−.007
Social Support from Family and Friends	−.137*	−.130	−.131	−.096

*$p < .05$
**$p < .01$
***$p < .0005$

TABLE 7.3 Changes in Infant Temperament and Nocturnal Sleep Patterns During the Postpartum ($N = 226$)

Variable	3 Weeks Postpartum	6 Weeks Postpartum	3 Months Postpartum	6 Months Postpartum	p
Infant Temperament [M, SD]					
Fussy–Difficult*	19.71 (4.88)	18.64 (4.69)	15.65 (4.43)	15.37 (4.08)	< .0005[a]
Unadaptable**	4.44 (2.20)	4.21 (2.18)	4.05 (1.97)	3.78 (1.95)	.002[c]
Dull***	2.41 (1.86)	2.71 (1.78)	2.31 (1.72)	2.31 (1.62)	.004[a]
Unpredictable****	8.97 (3.27)	8.21 (3.17)	7.09 (2.87)	6.58 (2.78)	< .0005[b]
Infant Nocturnal Sleep					
Sleeps Through Night [%]	2%	16%	57%	61%	< .0005[a]

[a]Difference between 3 weeks and 6 weeks, and 6 weeks and 3 months statistically significant.
[b]Differences between 3 weeks and 6 weeks, 6 weeks and 3 months, and 3 months and 6 months statistically significant.
[c]Difference between 3 and 6 months statistically significant.
*Potential range of scores = 6 to 42; higher scores indicate more difficult temperament.
**Potential range of scores = 2 to 14; higher scores indicate more difficult temperament.
***Potential range of scores = −5 to +13; higher scores indicate more difficult temperament.
****Potential range of scores = 3 to 21; higher scores indicate more difficult temperament.

TABLE 7.4   Correlations of Infant Temperament and Infant Nocturnal Sleep with Functional Status During the Postpartum (*N* = 226)

Variable	3 Weeks Postpartum Functional Status	6 Weeks Postpartum Functional Status	3 Months Postpartum Functional Status	6 Months Postpartum Functional Status
Infant Temperament				
Fussy–Difficult	−.160*	−.180**	−.078	−.151*
Unadaptable	−.148*	−.144*	−.150*	−.112
Dull	−.100	−.163*	−.053	−.107
Unpredictable	−.103	−.124	−.078	−.135*
Infant Nocturnal Sleep	.068	.080	.110	.024

*p < .05
**p < .01

and hindered them to continue their usual activities throughout the postpartum. We also looked at our data about the help the women received during the postpartum and their return to work following childbirth.

Changes in Psychological Symptoms

We first examined the data for each psychological symptom—feeling anxious, feeling depressed, and feeling better than usual (Table 7.1). More than one half (53%) of the women reported feeling anxious at three weeks after delivery; over one third (35%) reported this symptom at six weeks; slightly less than one quarter (24%) at three months; and almost one fifth (18%) at six months. Statistically significant changes ($p < .0005$) in feeling anxious were evident; the percentage of women who reported feeling anxious decreased from three weeks to six weeks, and from six weeks to three months postpartum. There was no evidence of a change from three to six months postpartum.

One quarter (25%) of the women reported feeling depressed at three weeks postpartum; the percentage dropped to approximately one fifth at six weeks (21%), three months (18%), and six months (18%). There was, however, no evidence of a statistically significant change in this symptom throughout the postpartum.

Approximately one quarter of the women reported feeling better than usual at three weeks (23%), six weeks (26%), and three months (27%) after delivery; the percentage dropped to slightly less than one fifth (18%) at six months. Again, there was no evidence of any statistically significant changes.

In response to our interview questions at six months postpartum, one fifth (19%) of the women told us that their emotional state hindered their adaptation during the postpartum. Some comments reflected feelings of anxiety. One woman simply stated that she was hindered in her adaptation by "anxiety." Another noted that she was "anxious about getting back to work."

Other comments from the women revealed variation in the length and intensity of depression. Commenting on the length of depression, one woman noted that she felt depressed for just two weeks. Conversely, another woman stated: "I still have depression. I had [depression] before but now [the feeling is] deeper and [lasts] longer." Commenting on the intensity of depression, one woman explained, "I did experience depression—it was mild, and I realized that had to be it. I am not one to sit around a lot but for about a week I did. It was the best week of my life because I didn't feel like doing anything and I didn't. And I realized it had to be depression." In contrast, another stated, "I was very depressed about the birth and stuff."

Still other comments reflected feelings of emotional lability. Examples of those comments are:

> Emotionally, I get my ups and downs.
> Emotionally, it is sometimes rocky.
> Emotionally, I have some days that are hard.

Elaborating, one women explained:

> There were a lot of emotional times. Someone would just look at me, and I thought I would just have to cry. [But] it passed quickly, and it wasn't something that lingered throughout the day. It was a spur of the moment type thing. [Overall,] we have been very happy.

Psychological Symptoms and Functional Status

The correlations between the three psychological symptoms—feeling anxious, feeling depressed, and feeling better than usual—and functional status ranged from very low to moderate in magnitude (Table 7.2). The negative relation between feeling anxious and functional status was statistically significant throughout the postpartum ($p < .05$); women who reported feeling anxious performed their usual activities at a lower level throughout the postpartum than did their counterparts who did not report feeling anxious. The negative relation between feeling depressed and functional status also was statistically significant throughout the postpartum ($p < .01$); those women who reported feeling depressed performed their usual activities at a lower level during the postpartum than did the women who did not report feeling depressed. None of the exceptionally low correlations between feeling better than usual and functional status reached statistical significance.

Changes in PSQ Psychosocial Health Variables

Examination of the PSQ scores for variables representing psychosocial health (gratification with labor and delivery, life satisfaction, satisfaction with motherhood, and maternal confidence in ability to cope with tasks of motherhood) revealed relatively positive evaluations, as well as some changes throughout the postpartum (Table 7.1). The woman's sense of gratification with her labor and delivery experience became more positive from three weeks to six weeks postpartum ($p < .0005$). Moreover, the woman's satisfaction with motherhood increased from six weeks to three months after delivery ($p = .024$). Furthermore, the woman's evaluation of her confidence in her ability to cope with the tasks of motherhood become progressively more positive from three weeks to six weeks to three months postpartum ($p < .0005$). No other changes in these variables were evident, nor were any changes evident in the woman's satisfaction with her life.

PSQ Psychosocial Health Variables and Functional Status

All of the correlations between the psychosocial health variables measured by the PSQ and functional status were low in magnitude (Table 7.2). Although the signs of the correlations are negative, the relations are positive because lower PSQ scores indicate positive evaluations (see Appendix). The positive relation between the woman's satisfaction with motherhood and her functional status was statistically significant throughout the postpartum ($p < .05$), as was the positive relation be-tween the woman's confidence in her ability to cope with the tasks of motherhood and functional status ($p < .05$). That is, greater satisfaction with motherhood and greater maternal confidence were associated with a higher level of performance of usual activities. The correlations of gratification with labor and delivery and life satisfaction with functional status were not statistically significant.

Changes in PSQ Family Relationships Variables

Examination of the PSQ scores for variables representing family rela-tionships revealed relatively positive evaluations (Table 7.1). The data revealed no evidence of changes in the women's evaluations of the quality of the marital relationship after delivery or social support from family and friends. In contrast, the women perceived that their husbands participated less in child care at six weeks than at three weeks postpar-tum ($p = .044$).

Family Relationships and Functional Status

The correlations between the family relationships variables from the PSQ—quality of the marital relationship after delivery, father participa-tion in child care, and support from family and friends—and functional status were exceptionally low in magnitude (Table 7.2). The positive relation between social support from family and friends and functional status was statistically significant only at three weeks postpartum ($p < .05$); greater support was associated with a higher level of performance of usual activities. The positive relation between quality of the marital relationship and functional status was statistically significant only at three months postpartum ($p < .01$); at that time, a rating of higher quality was associated with a higher level of performance of usual activities.

Help from Family and Friends

Throughout the postpartum, the women in our study reported that they received help for infant care, care of other children, housework, meal preparation, errands, and other household activities. Almost all

(98%) of the women had some help during the first three weeks after delivery. More than three quarters of those women received help from their husbands (79%) and/or from their mothers or mothers-in-law (77%). Very few (5%) women had paid help during the first three weeks of the postpartum.

More than four fifths (86%) of the women still had help by six weeks postpartum. Almost two thirds (63%) continued to receive help from their husbands. Just a few (4%) continued to receive help from their mothers or mothers-in-law. Almost one tenth (8%) had paid help by this time. More than one fifth (22%) relied on a combination of people.

More than four fifths (84%) of the women again had help at three months postpartum. Approximately two thirds (67%) of those women received help from their husbands; only few (3%) had help from their mothers or mothers-in-law. Slightly more than one tenth (11%) of the women had paid help at that time.

At six months after delivery, more than four fifths (86%) of the women still had help. Almost two thirds (61%) of those women received help from their husbands; just a few (5%) had help from their mothers or mothers-in-law. More than one eighth (14%) of the women had paid help.

Return to Work and Help With Child Care

Almost two thirds (65%) of the 20 women who returned to paid work by three weeks postpartum reported that they were the primary source of child care. For the most part, these women were either working out of their homes or had jobs that enabled them to bring their infants to the workplace. Other women relied on others for help with infant care as they began to return to work. The husbands, mothers, or mothers-in-law of one tenth of the women provided child care. Another one tenth of the women relied on an in-home baby sitter. The remainder used a combination of people for child care.

In contrast to the situation at three weeks postpartum, less than one tenth (7%) of the 41 women who returned to paid work by six weeks after delivery reported that they were the primary source of child care. The husbands, mothers, or mothers-in-law of more than one quarter (29%) of the women provided child care. One fifth (20%) employed in-home baby sitters. The same number relied on a combination of people for child care.

By three months postpartum, almost one fifth (17%) of the 97 women who by then returned to paid work reported that they were the primary source of child care. The husbands, mothers, or mothers-in-law of almost one third (29%) of the women provided child care. A friend or neighbor provided help for a few (6%) women. More than one eighth (14%) relied on an in-home baby sitter. Several women (17%) relied on day care or family care, that is, care of the infant by a person who provides care in his or her own home for a few children. Almost one fifth (18%) used a combination of people for child care.

At six months after childbirth, slightly more than one eighth (13%) of the 133 women who had by then returned to work reported that they were the primary source of child care. The husbands, mothers, or mothers-in-law of almost a third (30%) of the women provided child care. Almost one fifth (17%) relied on an in-home baby sitter, and the same number relied on a combination of people for child care. Another one fifth (19%) relied on day care or family care.

Help from Family and Friends and Functional Status

We examined our data to determine the extent to which having help during the time after delivery affected the women's performance of their usual activities. At six weeks postpartum, the women who had help had slightly lower ($M = 3.44$) functional status than those who did not have help ($M = 3.59$) ($p = .021$). There was no evidence of a relation between help and functional status at any other time during the postpartum.

When we interviewed the women in our study at six months after delivery, they enhanced our understanding of how the help they had from others both helped and hindered them with the continuation of their usual activities. Almost half (46%) of the women reported that their husbands were a major source of help during the postpartum. A typical comment was: "My husband was real supportive and very understanding." The women especially regarded the help their husbands gave them with household and child care as supportive. For example, one woman stated: "[My husband] gave me a lecture that I couldn't do anything. He took on a lot of responsibilities for the first month—I didn't do anything. He took care of the house and took care of everything." Another woman added, "[My husband] really loves [our daughter]. He will take her with him, or feed her, or watch her." Still another women commented, "[My husband] took off from work and helped me a lot the first week. He took turns getting up at night to take care of the baby, so I didn't have to do it all the time."

Almost one quarter (23%) of the women noted that family members were especially supportive. Mothers, mothers-in-law, sisters-in-law, and aunts were cited as particularly strong sources of support. Examples of the women's comments are: "My mother was a great help. She came home the first day and stayed the first evening." "For the first week I went to my mother-in-law's and [her] support got me back on my feet." "My sister in law has been tremendous." "I have an aunt who lives close by, and she helped me out a lot."

Another source of help during the postpartum was the women's friends. A few (6%) of the women cited a particular friend or group of friends who was supportive throughout the postpartum. The women's comments included: "One friend in particular has been amazing." "A couple of really good friends [were especially helpful.] Without them, I would not have been able to make it through. [I would not have been] able to talk and laugh and take care of [my baby]." "Having a lot of friends to talk to [was very helpful]."

Conversely, slightly less than one tenth (8%) of the women noted that family members and other people hindered their postpartum adaptation. Two women mentioned problems in their marital relationships. One woman's husband suffered from depression; she explained: "My husband has been suffering from depression and that has been hindering, because of some of his behavior to me and the children, and the baby. We are picking up on counseling." The other woman's husband was distressed by the birth of their twins; she stated: "We had a really rough time going through this. It came to the point of nearly separating when the twins were a couple of months old. He freaked out that we were having twins and [started] doing a lot of crazy stuff and wasn't around a lot."

Other women noted that their mothers or mothers-in-law created problems for them. One woman commented, "My mother made me crazy—everything I did was wrong. It made me totally sad." Another said, "[When] my mother-in-law was here and said negative things, I found them very hard."

Still other women pointed to the criticism they received from various people. One woman noted, "The people [who] badger me that I was not doing something right—that was stressful." Another added, "People did not give me time to rest; they didn't understand."

Changes in Infant Temperament and Functional Status

Maternal perception of infant temperament changed throughout the postpartum (Table 7.3). In particular, the women regarded their infants as becoming less fussy and difficult from three weeks to six weeks and from six weeks to three months after birth ($p < .0005$). In contrast, the women regarded their infants as becoming increasingly dull or placid from three to six weeks but less dull or placid from six weeks to three months after birth ($p = .004$). In addition, the women rated their infants as becoming progressively more predictable throughout the postpartum, with statistically significant changes from three weeks to six weeks to three months to six months ($p < .0005$). Finally, the women rated their infants as becoming more adaptable over the first six months of life ($p = .002$), with statistically significant changes between three and six months postpartum ($p = .025$).

The correlations between infant temperament and functional status were of exceptionally low magnitude (Table 7.4). However, some statistically significant correlations were evident. The greater the woman's perception of her infant's unadaptability, the lower the level of her performance of usual activities at three weeks, six weeks, and three months after delivery ($p < .05$). Furthermore, the greater the woman's perception of fussiness of her infant, the lower the level of her performance of usual activities at three weeks, six weeks, and six months postpartum ($p < .05$). Moreover, the greater the woman's perception of infant dullness or placidness, the lower the level of her performance of usual activities at six weeks after delivery ($p < .05$). In addition, the greater the woman's perception of infant unpredictability, the lower the level of her performance of usual activities at six months postpartum ($p < .05$).

Changes in Infant Nocturnal Sleep Patterns and Functional Status

As can be seen in Table 7.3, very few (2%) infants slept through the night at three weeks postpartum. However, the percentage steadily increased to close to one fifth (16%) at six weeks, more than one half (57%) at three months, and close to two thirds (61%) at six months. These changes were statistically significant for three weeks to six weeks and from six weeks to three months ($p < .0005$). The correlations between infant nocturnal sleep and functional status were of exceptionally low magnitude and none were statistically significant (Table 7.4).

CONCLUSION

Our data indicate that some changes occurred in women's psychosocial health, family relationships, and functional status during the first six postpartum months. More specifically, changes in occurred in some but not all of the variables we selected to represent the self-concept and interdependence adaptation modes, in response to the focal stimulus of the postpartum. These data provide some support for the Roy Adaptation Model proposition asserting that changes in the focal stimulus are related to changes in adaptation responses. The findings, however, yielded a more parsimonious version of the portion of our Theory of Adaptation During Childbearing addressing psychosocial health and family relationships than we originally proposed.

Our finding of changes in the psychological symptom of feeling anxious during the first six postpartum months is in keeping with the results of other studies (Gjerdingen & Chaloner, 1994b; Singh & Sexena, 1991) and with our findings for this symptom during pregnancy (see chapter 4, Table 4.1). Our data did not, however, permit us to determine the level of anxiety experienced by the women in our study.

Of interest is the finding of no evidence of changes in women's reports of the psychological symptom of feeling depressed throughout the postpartum. Although the percentage of women in our study who reported feeling depressed (see Table 7.1) is within the 3% to 27% range reported by Bryan and colleagues (1999), we did not find any evidence of the changes in depression throughout the postpartum reported by other investigators (Gjerdingen, Froberg, & Kochevar, 1991; Affonso et al., 1993). Also of interest is that we found no evidence of changes in the women's reports of feeling depressed during the three trimesters of pregnancy (see chapter 4, Table 4.1).

Our postpartum findings for the psychological symptom of feeling better than usual conflict with our findings for pregnancy. More women reported feeling better than usual during the second trimester of pregnancy than during the first or third trimesters (see chapter 4, Table 4.1). In contrast, there was no evidence of statistically significant changes in this symptom during the postpartum. Thus, our speculation that this psychological symptom would vary as the postpartum progressed was not substantiated.

Our findings of relatively positive evaluations of the aspects of psychosocial health included in the PSQ during the first six postpartum months are in keeping with results of other studies (Halman, Oakley, & Lederman, 1995; Reece & Harkless, 1998; Sampselle et al., 1999; Weiss, 1991). Furthermore, our finding of progressively greater maternal confidence in ability to cope with tasks of motherhood from three weeks to three months postpartum is in keeping with the findings of our earlier study (Tulman, Fawcett, Groblewski, & Silverman, 1990), as well as with the direction of Lederman and Lederman's (1987) finding of greater maternal confidence at six weeks than at three days after delivery. In addition, our finding of no changes in life satisfaction in our present study is consistent with our finding for this variable in our earlier study (Tulman, Fawcett, Groblewski, & Silverman, 1990). In contrast, our present study finding of greater gratification with labor and delivery at six weeks than at three weeks postpartum conflicts with the finding of no change in this variable in our earlier study (Tulman, Fawcett, Groblewski, & Silverman, 1990).

Our finding of a more positive evaluation of the father's participation in child care at three weeks than at six weeks postpartum is in keeping with Lederman and Lederman's (1987) finding of greater dissatisfaction with father participation at six weeks than at three weeks after delivery but conflicts with our earlier finding of no changes in father participation (Tulman, Fawcett, Groblewski, & Silverman, 1990). Our finding of no changes in social support from family and friends throughout the postpartum also conflicts with other investigators' findings of changes in social support during the postpartum (Gjerdingen & Chaloner, 1994a; Lederman & Lederman, 1987; McVeigh, 2000b; Mercer & Ferketich, 1995) and in the findings of our earlier study (Tulman, Fawcett, Groblewski, & Silverman, 1990). Similarly, our finding of no changes in the quality of the marital relationship after delivery conflicts with the results of other studies, which revealed that greater dissatisfaction with the marital relationship at six weeks than at three days (Lederman & Lederman, 1987; Mercer, Ferketich, & DeJoseph, 1993). This finding is, however, consistent with the results of our earlier study (Tulman, Fawcett, Groblewski, & Silverman, 1990).

The direction of changes in the fussy-difficult, dull, unadaptable, and unpredictable aspects of infant temperament (Table 7.3) are similar to the findings of another study (Gennaro, Tulman, & Fawcett, 1990). These findings add to the evidence of changes in the direction of less difficult temperament as the infant matures (Koniak-Griffin & Ludington-Hoe, 1988; Vaughn, Deinard, & Egelund, 1980).

The statistically significant correlations between some variables representing the Roy Adaptation Model self-concept response mode and the role function response mode variable of functional status (Table 7.2) indicate that these modes are interrelated components of adaptation during the postpartum. The lack of statistical support for the association between some self-concept mode variables and functional status indicates that this portion our Theory of Adaptation During Childbearing is more parsimonious than originally proposed. Furthermore, the magnitude of the statistically significant correlations indicates that the relation between the two modes is moderate at best (Table 7.2). These findings, together with our findings for pregnancy (chapter 4), clarify the relation between self-concept and role function mode responses reported by Chiou (2000).

Our findings of statistically significant correlations between feeling anxious and functional status, and feeling depressed and functional status, add to the limited empirical evidence available about the association between psychological symptoms and performance of usual activities during the postpartum. Our data do not, however, permit us to determine whether psychological symptoms influence functional status or vice versa. Moreover, our data do not permit us to determine whether the association between psychological symptoms and functional status might be reciprocal, such that an increase in anxiety, for example, results in a decrease in functional status, and the decrease in functional status results in a further increase in anxiety.

The finding of just two statistically significant correlations between PSQ family relationships variables and functional status (Table 7.2), an inconsistent pattern of statistically significant correlations between aspects of infant temperament and functional status (Table 7.4), and no evidence of statistically significant correlations between infant nocturnal sleep and functional status (Table 7.4), added to the lack of any statistically significant correlations for family relationships variables and functional status during pregnancy (chapter 4), collectively provide minimal support for a relation between the Roy Adaptation Model interdependence and role function response modes and minimal support for that portion of our Theory of Adaptation During Childbearing. These findings conflict with the results of Chiou's (2000) meta-analysis, which revealed an association between interdependence and role function mode variables in four studies.

Our finding that the women in our study reported that their husbands were a major source of help in their adaptation during childbearing is in keeping with other investigators' findings that husbands are the principal source of social support for a woman following delivery (Isabella & Isabella, 1994; Lederman & Lederman, 1987). Furthermore, our finding that the women's mothers were an additional source of help is in keeping with Isabella and Isabella's (1994) study results. Of particular note is that husbands, mothers, and mothers-in-law were primary sources of child care in almost a third of cases at three and six months, the time when women in our study were likely to return to work. Having help was not, however, strongly or consistently related to the women's postpartum functional status.

REFERENCES

Affonso, D. D., De, A. K., Horowitz, J. A., & Mayberry, L. J. (2000). An international study exploring levels of postpartum depressive symptomatology. *Journal of Psychosomatic Research, 49*, 207–216.

Affonso, D. D., Lovett, S., Paul, S. M., & Sheptak, S. (1990). A standardized interview that differentiates pregnancy and postpartum symptoms from perinatal clinical depression. *Birth, 17*, 121–130.

Affonso, D., Mayberry, L., Lovett, S., Paul, S., Johnson, B., Nussbaum, R., & Newman, L. (1993). Pregnancy and postpartum depressive symptoms. *Journal of Women's Health, 2*, 157–164.

Allen, H. (1999). "How was it for you?" Debriefing for postnatal women: Does it help? *Professional Care of Mother and Child, 9*(3), 77–79.

Bates, J. E. (1987). Temperament in infancy. In J. D. Osofsky (Ed.), *Handbook of infant development* (2nd ed., pp. 1101–1149). New York: Wiley.

Bates, J. E., Freeland, C. A. B., & Lounsbury, M. L. (1979). Measurement of infant difficultness. *Child Development, 50*, 794–803.

Beck, C. T. (1991). Maternity blues research: A critical review. *Issues in Mental Health Nursing, 12*, 291–300.

Beck, C. T. (1999). Postpartum depression: Stopping the thief that steals motherhood. *AWHONN Lifelines, 3*(4), 41–44.

Beck, C. T., Reynolds, M. A., & Rutowski, P. (1992). Maternity blues and postpartum depression. *Journal of Obstetric, Gynecologic, and Neonatal Nursing, 21*, 287–293.

Bergant, A. M., Heim, K., Ulmer, H., & Illmensee, K. (1999). Early postnatal depressive mood: Association with obstetric and psychosocial factors. *Journal of Psychosomatic Research, 46*, 391–394.

Bryan, T. L., Georgiopoulos, A. M., Harms, R. W., Huxsahl, J. E., Larson, D. R., & Yawn, B. P. (1999). Incidence of postpartum depression in Olmsted County, Minnesota: A population based, retrospective study. *Journal of Reproductive Medicine, 44*, 351–358.

Carey, W. B. (1983). Some pitfalls in infant temperament research. *Infant Behavior and Development, 6*, 247–254.

Chiou, C-P. (2000). A meta-analysis of the interrelationships between the modes in Roy's adaptation model. *Nursing Science Quarterly, 13,* 252–258.

Darling-Fisher, C. S. (1987). *The relationship between mothers' and fathers' Eriksonian psychosocial attributes, perceptions of family support, and adaptation to parenthood.* Unpublished doctoral dissertation, University of Michigan, Ann Arbor.

Drake, M. L., Verhulst, D., & Fawcett, J. (1988). Physical and psychological symptoms experienced by Canadian women and their husbands during pregnancy and the postpartum. *Journal of Advanced Nursing, 13,* 436–440.

Fawcett, J., & York, R. (1986). Spouses' physical and psychological symptoms during pregnancy and the postpartum. *Nursing Research, 35,* 144–148.

Fishbein, E. G., & Burggraf, E. (1998). Early postpartum discharge: How are mothers managing? *Journal of Obstetric, Gynecologic, and Neonatal Nursing, 27,* 142–148.

Gennaro, S. (1988). Postpartal anxiety and depression in mothers of term and preterm infants. *Nursing Research, 37,* 82–85.

Gennaro, S., Tulman, L., & Fawcett, J. (1990). Temperament in preterm and full-term infants at three and six months of age. *Merrill-Palmer Quarterly, 36,* 201–215.

Gjerdingen, D. K., & Chaloner, K. (1994a). Mothers' experience with household roles and social support during the first postpartum year. *Women and Health, 21*(4), 57–74.

Gjerdingen, D. K., & Chaloner, K. (1994b). The relationship of women's postpartum mental health to employment, childbirth, and social support. *Journal of Family Practice, 38,* 465–472.

Gjerdingen, D. K., Froberg, D. G., & Fontaine, P. (1990). A causal model describing the relationship of women's postpartum health to social support, length of leave, and complications of childbirth. *Women and Health, 16,* 71–87.

Gjerdingen, D. K., Froberg, D. G., & Kochevar, L. (1991). Changes in women's mental and physical health from pregnancy through six months postpartum. *Journal of Family Practice, 32,* 161–166.

Gotlib, I. H., Wiffen, V. E., Mount, J. H., Milne, K., & Cordy, N. I. (1989). Prevalence rates and demographic characteristics associated with depression in pregnancy and the postpartum. *Journal of Consulting and Clinical Psychology, 57,* 269–274.

Halman, L. J., Oakley, D., & Lederman, R. (1995). Adaptation to pregnancy and motherhood among subfecund and fecund primiparous women. *Maternal-Child Nursing Journal, 23,* 90–100.

Harris, B., Lovett, L., Newcombe, R. G., Read, G. F., Walker, R., & Riad-Fahmy, D. (1994). Maternity blues and major endocrine changes: Cardiff puerperal mood and hormone study II. *British Medical Journal, 308,* 949–953.

Hubert, N. C., & Wachs, T. D. (1985). Parental perceptions of the behavioral components of infant easiness/difficultness. *Child Development, 56,* 1525–1537.

Hubert, N. C., Wachs, T. D., Peters-Martin, P., & Gandour, M. J. (1982). The study of early temperament: Measurement and conceptual issues. *Child Development, 53,* 571–600.

Hughes, P. M., Turton, P., & Evans, C. D. H. (1999). Stillbirth as risk factor for depression and anxiety in the subsequent pregnancy: Cohort study. *British Medical Journal, 318,* 1721–1724.

Isabella, P. H., & Isabella, R. A. (1994). Correlates of successful breastfeeding: A study of social personal factors. *Journal of Human Lactation, 10,* 257–264.

Koenigseder, L. A. (1991). *Patterns of change in primiparas' moods and functional status: An extension of Rubin's nursing model.* Unpublished doctoral dissertation, University of Texas at Austin.

Koniak-Griffin, D., & Ludington-Hoe, S. M. (1988). Developmental and tempera- ment outcomes of sensory stimulation in healthy infants. *Nursing Research, 37,* 70–76.

Lederman, R. P., & Lederman, E. (1987). Dimensions of postpartum adaptation: Comparisons of multiparas 3 days and 6 weeks after delivery. *Journal of Psychoso- matic Obstetrics and Gynecology, 7,* 193–203.

Lederman, R. P., Weingarten, C-G. T., & Lederman, E. (1981). Postpartum Self- Evaluation Questionnaire: Measures of maternal adaptation. In R. P. Lederman, B. S. Raff, & P. Carroll (Eds.), *Perinatal parental behavior: Nursing research and implications for newborn health* (Birth Defects: Original Article Series, Vol. 17, No. 6, pp. 201–231). New York: March of Dimes Birth Defects Foundation.

Martin, L. L., & Reeder, S. J. (1991). *Essentials of maternity nursing: Family-centered care.* Philadelphia: Lippincott.

McVeigh, C. (1997a). An Australian study of functional status after childbirth. *Midwifery, 13,* 172–178.

McVeigh, C. (1997b). Functional status after childbirth: A comparison of Australian women from English and non-English speaking backgrounds. *Australian College of Midwives Incorporated Journal, 10*(2), 15–21.

McVeigh, C. A. (2000a). Anxiety and functional status after childbirth. *Australian College of Midwives Incorporated Journal, 13*(1), 14–18.

McVeigh, C. A. (2000b). Investigating the relationship between satisfaction with social support and functional status after childbirth. *MCN: American Journal of Maternal Child Nursing, 25,* 25–30.

Mercer, R. T. (1995). *Becoming a mother: Research on maternal identity from Rubin to the present.* New York: Springer Publishing.

Mercer, R. T., & Ferketich, S. L. (1994). Predictors of maternal role competence by risk status. *Nursing Research, 43,* 38–43.

Mercer, R. T., & Ferketich, S. L. (1995). Experienced and inexperienced mothers' maternal competence during infancy. *Research in Nursing and Health, 18,* 333–343.

Mercer, R. T., Ferketich, S. L., & DeJoseph, J. F. (1993). Predictors of partner relationships during pregnancy and infancy. *Research in Nursing and Health, 16,* 45–56.

Murata, A., Nadaoka, T., Morioka, Y., Oiji, A., & Saito, H. (1998). Prevalence and background factors of maternity blues. *Gynecological and Obstetric Investigation, 46,* 99–104.

Norbeck, J. S., & Tilden, V. P. (1983). Life stress, social support, and emotional disequilibrium in complications of pregnancy: A prospective, multivariate study. *Journal of Health and Social Behavior, 24,* 30–46.

O'Hara, M. W. (1986). Social support, life events, and depression during pregnancy and the puerperium. *Archives of General Psychiatry, 43,* 569–573.

O'Hara, M. W., & Swain, A. M. (1996). Rates and risk of postpartum depression: A meta-analysis. *International Review of Psychiatry, 8*, 37–54.

Oshio, S. (1992). *Mother's mental representation of her infant and its effect on infant organization and mother's perception of self.* Unpublished doctoral dissertation, University of Washington, Seattle.

Parisher, S. F., Nasrallah, H. A., & Gardner, D. K. (1997). Postpartum mood disorders: Clinical perspectives. *Journal of Women's Health, 6*, 421–434.

Pitt, B. (1973). Maternity blues. *British Journal of Psychiatry, 122*, 431–433.

Reece, S. M., & Harkless, G. (1998). Self-efficacy, stress, and parental adaptation: Applications to the care of childbearing families. *Journal of Family Nursing, 4*, 198–215.

Reeder, S. J., Martin, L. L., & Koniak-Griffin, D. (1997). *Maternity nursing: Family, newborn, and women's health care* (18th ed.). Philadelphia: Lippincott-Raven.

Ruchala, P. L., & Halstead, L. (1994). The postpartum experience of low-risk women: A time of adjustment and change. *Maternal-Child Nursing Journal, 22*, 83–89.

Sampselle, C. M., Seng, J., Yeo, S., Killion, C., & Oakley, D. (1999). Physical activity and postpartum well-being. *Journal of Obstetric, Gynecologic, and Neonatal Nursing, 28*, 41–49.

Singh, U., & Sexena, M. (1991). Anxiety during pregnancy and after birth. *Psychological Studies, 36*, 108–111.

Thomas, A., Chess, S., & Birch, H. G. (1968). *Temperament and behavior disorders in children.* New York: New York University Press.

Thomas, A., Chess, S., & Korn, S. J. (1982). The reality of difficult temperament. *Merrill-Palmer Quarterly, 28*, 1–20.

Tulman, L., Fawcett, J., Groblewski, L., & Silverman, L. (1990). Changes in functional status after childbirth. *Nursing Research, 39*, 70–75.

Vaughn, B., Deinard, A., & Egeland, B. (1980). Measuring temperament in pediatric practice. *Journal of Pediatrics, 96*, 510–514.

Weiss, M.E. (1991). The relationship between marital interdependence and adaptation to parenthood in primiparous couples. *Dissertation Abstracts International, 51*, 3783B.

Whiffen, V. E., & Gotlib, I. H. (1993). Comparison of postpartum and nonpostpartum depression: Clinical presentation, psychiatric history, and psychosocial functioning. *Journal of Consulting and Clinical Psychology, 61*, 485–494.

Wolman, W. L., Chalmers, B., Hofmeyr, G. J., & Nikodem, V. C. (1993). Postpartum depression and companionship in the clinical birth environment: A randomized, controlled study. *American Journal of Obstetrics and Gynecology, 168*, 1388–1393.

Part IV

WHAT WOMEN NEED DURING THE CHILDBEARING PERIOD

8

Looking Back at Childbearing: Women's Expectations and Recommendations

We regard pregnancy and the postpartum as times of considerable and often profound change to which women adapt in various ways. At six months postpartum, we asked the women who participated in our study to reflect back on the pregnancy and postpartum and compare the experience with their expectations. Their responses underscored the need to advise every woman that the childbearing experience is rarely what she expects it to be. In this chapter, we present our analysis of the women's recollections of their childbearing experiences, along with their recommendations for lifestyle adjustments that can facilitate adaptation during pregnancy and the postpartum.

REFLECTIONS ABOUT PREGNANCY

Reflecting back on their pregnancies, women varied in how their experiences compared with their expectations. Only a few (2%) of the women stated that they had no expectations about their pregnancies. One woman noted, "I purposely did not have a lot of expectations because I did not want to be disappointed."

More than one quarter (29%) of the women in our study indicated that their pregnancies met their expectations. A multipara explained, "I think [this pregnancy] compared closely [to what I expected], probably because I had already been pregnant before and I knew what to expect. I didn't have any problems."

Slightly more than one quarter (27%) of the women indicated that their pregnancies were easier than expected. One woman commented, "It was better than what I expected. I had no problems—it was a great pregnancy and a great delivery." Elaborating, another women stated:

> It was great; it was a lot easier [then I had expected]. It made a huge difference not having a stressful job. I was happy, and I was doing things that made me

happy, and I was on my own schedule, so if I was tired, I could do what I needed to do. I expected it to be more restricted, but it wasn't. That is because I did not have to do something I did not want to do. If you are psychologically happy during pregnancy, I think you are happy all the way through. What I expected was to be going to work and having a large part of my day being rigid as far as what you had to be doing, and I expected to be more exhausted.

Conversely, two fifths (40%) of the women stated that their pregnancies were harder than expected. One woman commented, "It was more difficult [than] my first pregnancy. With this one, I couldn't move; I felt real tired." Another woman explained:

I was sicker and more tired than I thought [I would be]. I guess I thought pregnancy would go a long naturally [but] I never got it together. I didn't have a lot of expectations because I was the first [of] my family and my friends to get pregnant. I had never known any pregnant women; it was new.

A few (3%) other women found the pregnancy both harder and easier than expected. Representative comments were:

I think it was what I expected. [But] I was more tired, and I didn't expect that—I was surprised about that.

It was slightly different than my first pregnancy. I had a lot [more] Braxton-Hicks contractions in the third trimester than I expected, but in all other ways it was easier than I thought it would be.

REFLECTIONS ABOUT THE POSTPARTUM

In reflecting back on the time since delivery from the vantage point of six months postpartum, just a few (3%) of the women stated that they had no expectations. One woman noted, "Since the delivery, I don't know. I didn't have any expectations. I have taken things one day at a time." Another commented, "I didn't know what to expect. Everything worked itself out, especially with the help that I had."

One sixth (17%) of the women in our study indicated that their first six months postpartum went about as expected. One multipara commented, "[Things] are pretty much what I expected—pretty much the same compared to the other ones." Another women explained:

It is pretty much what I expected—constant moving. I never stop. I went back to work. Everything is back to normal, like before I was pregnant. We might not socialize as much but we go out.

Another one sixth (17%) of the women indicated that this time period had been easier and better than they had expected. One woman explained:

> I am trying to remember. I think it went better [than I had expected]. I thought I would have trouble getting started and running my day. I expected to be bouncing off the walls but with the help of an agreeable baby, I have been able to work out my life. I feel really good about it. I have a lot of potential time. I can stop and do things.

In contrast, more than one half (52%) of the women stated that the first six months postpartum were harder than they had expected. One woman, for example, ascribed her difficulty during the postpartum to the baby's illness. She stated, "[The months since delivery] were rougher than I thought. Because of the baby's ear infections. I was [always] wondering if he was okay or not."

Another woman attributed the difficulty to changes in her social life with her husband. She explained, "I like the baby and staying home but my husband was used to going to the clubs and going out, and we really don't do it that much anymore. We can't do the same things that we did before because of the money."

Another woman attributed the difficulty to the balance between income from part-time work and the cost of child care, as well as her own reluctance to have another person care for her baby. She said:

> I thought I would be back to work, and I haven't. Back to work to me was only part time. I was only working 10 to 12 hours a week. Even that amount of time is difficult because of the child care problem and my husband working and traveling. [A salary of] $5.00 an hour at 12 hours a week was hardly worth the aggravation to find a sitter and paying a sitter. I thought I would want to get out of the house, but I don't mind not getting out of the house. I did not anticipate being so leery about leaving her with people. I thought it would be easier psychologically than it has been. I am paranoid about giving her to someone else to watch. . . . It really keeps you home. Trying to go places with her is difficult.

A few (2%) women found that the postpartum was both harder and easier than they had expected. Speaking for the others, one woman explained:

> I think it was harder and easier. I expected it to be really hard dealing with two, but it is easier, but harder. In some ways, I already know how to take

care of a baby so that's easier, but it is harder to take care of two and give so much attention to two. More energy than I expected. I get a lot more done.

THE WOMEN'S RECOMMENDATIONS

When asked, "If you were to have another child, what (if anything) would you do differently during your pregnancy or after the birth of the baby to help your recovery?" approximately one quarter (24%) of the women stated that they would do nothing different. Some of those women simply answered "Nothing."

Others elaborated; for example, one woman commented, "I don't think I would do anything [different]. I am happy with the way they went." Another woman noted, "I don't know if I would do things different. I feel pretty happy with how things are going." Still another woman stated, "That is my way of life, and that is what I knew. I don't see where it would be any different."

The remaining three quarters (76%) of the women maintained that they would do something different. Their recommendations are listed in Table 8.1.

The most frequently cited recommendations were to be in better shape before another pregnancy (more than one third of the women

TABLE 8.1   What Women Would Do Differently (*N* = 173)

Recommendations	Percentage*
Be in better shape before another pregnancy	36%
Have extra household and/or child care help	33%
Take a longer maternity leave from work	16%
Take better care of self during the pregnancy and postpartum	14%
Try to get more rest	10%
Adjust work or school schedule	9%
Do less during recovery	9%
Have different childbirth conditions	8%
Have more realistic expectations	7%
Space children differently	5%
Select a different infant feeding method	4%
Develop a better support system	4%
Have more money	2%
Continue to work	1%

*Exceeds 100% because some women gave more than one response.

made this recommendation) and to have extra household and/or child care help (one third of the women made this recommendation). Comments from women who recommended being in better shape before another pregnancy included:

> I would try to get into good eating habits.
>
> I would exercise more.
>
> Maybe stay more active during my pregnancy to help with less weight gain.

Examples of comments from women who recommended extra household and/or child care help were:

> If I could afford it, I would get someone to clean for a month or two.
>
> I would get someone to come over so I could take my naps in the afternoon.

CONCLUSION

Although most women found their pregnancies to have been about the same or easier than expected, a substantial minority found their pregnancies to be more difficult. Furthermore, the majority of the women found the six months after delivery to have been more difficult than what they had expected due to a variety of factors. The vast majority of women thought that they would try to do at least one thing differently if they were to have another child. These findings closely follow the qualitative findings from one of our earlier studies (Tulman & Fawcett, 1991). The women's recommendations also point to interventions that women may wish to try before conception ("being in better shape," "more realistic expectations," "spacing of children," "developing support system," "more money"), during pregnancy and delivery ("better care of self," "childbirth conditions") and during the postpartum ("more help," "longer maternity leave," "more rest"). Their recommendations also tell us that counseling of pregnant and postpartum women should include information about the variability of women's responses to pregnancy and new motherhood.

REFERENCE

Tulman, L., & Fawcett, J. (1991) Recovery from childbirth: Looking back 6 months after delivery. *Health Care for Women International, 12,* 341–350.

9

Recommendations for
Practice and Policy

Our study results certainly support Gottesman's (1992) statement that "Pregnancy is an intense preparatory period of the mind as well as of the body for motherhood" (p. 108). Our study results also support Newton's (1955) claim that women "experience pregnancy *emotionally* as well as *physically*" (p. 28). The postpartum also is an intense period, a time of considerable turmoil for some women, and a time of adjustment for all women. Mercer (1995) pointed out that the events surrounding childbirth threaten the woman's self image, body image, and ideal image. Elaborating, she stated, "[The woman's] major concerns are her ability to function within the norms established by others before her, to maintain control of her body and behavior and situations within her control, and to survive the experience intact" (p. 128). Our study results point the way to the particular aspects of both the woman's physical health and her psychosocial health that require attention during pregnancy and the postpartum. As Gottesman (1992) pointed out, "Appreciation of the complex nature of the preparatory work of pregnancy will lead to sensitive and individualized prenatal care that nurtures the psychological as well as the physical gestation of mother and child" (p. 108). And, as Newton (1955) noted, women need "watching and perhaps a little help" both emotionally and physically (p. 28) during pregnancy and the postpartum.

Our suggestions for interventions are consistent with the Roy Adaptation Model nursing process, which emphasizes active participation of the patient in assessment, goal setting, and intervention (Roy, 1984; Roy & Andrews, 1999). Accordingly, we advocate active participation of the woman in discussions with a nurse or other health care professional to determine the optimal level of her functional status, to set goals for adaptation, and to identify strategies that will maintain or enhance her adaptation during pregnancy and the postpartum.

We agree with Newton's (1955) classic recommendations for attention to the selection of an appropriate time and place for discussions of the woman's experience of childbearing. We have found that women are quite willing and even eager to discuss their experiences throughout their pregnancies and the first six months postpartum. We collected our study data in the privacy of the women's homes, which may have been especially conducive to their willingness to share their experiences with us. An alternative to the woman's home is the clinician's office or the prenatal or postpartum clinic, provided that a quiet and private place can be found.

We also agree with Newton (1955) that "A mutual feeling of respect, trust, and goodwill is perhaps the most important of all in establishing the free expression of feelings" (p. 107). Building the respect, trust, and goodwill that are necessary for effective rapport may require more than one encounter between the woman and a health care professional. Accordingly, the health care professional should anticipate that the woman's active participation in a comprehensive assessment, goal setting, and interventions will occur over a period of time.

Our study results revealed that functional status changes over the three trimesters of pregnancy and the weeks and months postpartum, which indicate that each woman's functional status should be closely monitored. In addition, our study results revealed that certain physical health, psychosocial health, and family relationship variables change over the course of pregnancy and the weeks and months postpartum. These results indicate that physical symptoms, as well psychological symptoms and other psychosocial health and family relationship variables, also should be closely monitored.

Functional status can be monitored easily by means of the *Inventory of Functional Status–Antepartum Period* (IFSAP) (Fawcett, Tulman, & Myers, 1988) and the *Inventory of Functional Status After Childbirth* (IFSAC) (Tulman et al., 1991). Both questionnaires may be used to assess functional status by means of each woman's self-ratings, which could be done at home or in the health care professional's office waiting room. Alternatively, the nurse or other health care professional can use the IFSAP and IFSAC as structured interview guides. Either assessment format provides an opportunity for the woman to reflect on the impact of her childbearing experience on performance of her usual activities. Discussion between the health care professional and the woman can then focus on identification of interventions that will promote the woman's desired level of functional status throughout pregnancy and the postpartum. Specific recommendations to maintain, increase, or decrease the level performance of usual activities will, therefore, be based on each woman's standards, rather than an arbitrary standard set by the health care professional.

Our study results indicated that women may need help with their usual activities throughout pregnancy and the entire postpartum period. Even with help, many women did not experience full functional status during pregnancy, especially during the first and third trimester, and some women did not attain full functional status by six months after delivery. Discussions with each woman throughout pregnancy and the postpartum should focus on her desired level of functional status, because full functional status may not be a goal for some women. Women may want to maintain the current level, or increase or decrease their performance of usual activities at various times during pregnancy and the postpartum. Once a goal for level of functional status is established, discussion should focus on identification of strategies that will enable the woman to achieve her goal. Regardless of the goal, women should be counseled to avoid trying to be "superwomen" or "supermoms." Indeed, some women recommended having more realistic expectations about just what can be accomplished during pregnancy and the postpartum (see Table 8.1).

Although we found no statistical association between the woman's relationship with her husband or with her mother and functional status during pregnancy (chapter 4), and no association between social support from family and friends and functional status during the postpartum (chapter 7), some women commented that direct assistance and encouragement from their husband or mother or a friend helped them to continue their usual activities. Furthermore, many women recommended having extra household and/or child care help, and a few women recommended the development of a better support system (see Table 8.1). These findings underscore the need to encourage women to ask for help and to recognize that such help may facilitate achievement of their desired level of functional status.

Having help, however, was not always a positive experience for the women in our study. Indeed, some women told us that help from some family members and friends created problems or conflicts. Clearly, women need to be counseled to seek help from family members and friends, but to feel comfortable rejecting help when it is not supportive of their adaptation during the postpartum.

Physical and psychological symptoms can be monitored easily by use of the *Symptoms Checklist* (Fawcett & York, 1986). This instrument, like the IFSAP and IFSAC, can be used for the woman's self-rating or as an interview guide. Alternatively, instruments that measure specific symptoms can be used. For example, the *Postpartum Depression Screening Scale*

(Beck & Gable, 2000, 2001) can be used to monitor symptoms of postpartum depression. Physical energy can be monitored very easily by our one-item *Physical Energy Scale* (see Appendix).

Although our results revealed a minimal association between physical symptoms and functional status (chapters 2 and 5), the symptoms certainly should be actively treated, using any number of interventions given in nursing and obstetrics textbooks. In light of Mayberry's (1992) finding of greater symptom distress during the third trimester of pregnancy than six to eight weeks after delivery, special attention should be given to monitoring and treating physical symptoms during pregnancy. Furthermore, although we found little association between psychological symptoms and functional status, any interventions that result in a reduction in the anxiety and depression experienced by women during pregnancy and the postpartum, along with any interventions that promote feeling better than usual, are important to the woman's quality of life.

In light of our finding of an association between physical energy and functional status (see chapters 2 and 5), discussions should focus on ways each woman can maintain or increase her physical energy. The women's own recommendations in this regard center on doing less during the postpartum and trying to get more rest (see Table 8.1). Women may be able to follow those recommendations if they are able to have extra help with their household and child care activities, and if they are able to adjust their work or school schedule (see Table 8.1).

Clearly, women need to be encouraged to get more rest throughout the childbearing period, especially during the postpartum. Nurses and other health care professionals need to participate with women in creative problem-solving to find ways to adjust the women's work or school schedule to do less during the early months of the postpartum. Nurses also should seek opportunities to explain to members of the woman's family, especially her partner, how helpful and supportive they can be and encourage them to continue to offer their help and support after the immediate postpartum period. Noteworthy, however, is McVeigh and colleagues' (2002) finding that just 1.5% of the new fathers in their study increased their involvement in household activities and none increased their involvement in child care activities at six weeks postpartum. We concur with their recommendation that health care professionals encourage couples to negotiate the division of household and child care activities prior to the birth of the baby.

More than one half of the women in our study emphasized the need to be in better shape prior to pregnancy and/or to take better care of themselves during the pregnancy and postpartum. Eating properly and exercising are two ways in which any woman can take better care of herself at any time in life and, therefore, be in "better shape" prior to a pregnancy.

Eating properly and exercising also are ways in which women can control their weight gain or weight loss. The data we presented in chapter 3 indicate that women who gain more than their recommended weight for Body Mass Index category should be cautioned that they may experience a decrease in functional status during the third trimester of pregnancy. In addition, although we found little evidence of a statistical association between postpartum weight and functional status, more than one fifth of the women in our study pointed out that their weight hindered their performance of usual activities following delivery (chapter 6). Nurses should, therefore, assess women who are gaining weight at above the recommended levels for their prepregnant weight or are retaining excess weight during the postpartum, to determine whether functional status is diminished. Although dieting is not recommended during pregnancy or when breastfeeding, evaluation of the woman's nutrient intake may identify areas that require adjustment.

Various psychosocial and family relationship variables can be monitored with the *Prenatal Self-Evaluation Questionnaire* (PNSQ) (Lederman, 1984, 1996; Lederman, Lederman, Work, & McCann, 1979) and the *Postpartum Self-Evaluation Questionnaire* (PSQ) (Lederman, Weingarten, & Lederman, 1981). Those questionnaires certainly could be used as self-rating scales or interview guides.

Alternatively, less complex one-item questionnaires could be used to monitor changes in such variables as acceptance of pregnancy, satisfaction with motherhood, and father participation in child care. For example, the woman could be asked, "On a scale of 1 to 5, with 1 as lowest and 5 as highest, how satisfied are you with motherhood?" Sagrestano and colleagues (2002) found that single-item questionnaires are satisfactory alternatives to longer, standardized instruments for monitoring such variables as anxiety, depression, and social support.

Our study results revealed relatively positive evaluations of all variables measured by the PNSQ (chapter 4) and the PSQ (chapter 7), along with low but some statistically significant correlations between those variables and functional status. Accordingly, interventions should be directed to maintaining or increasing those positive evaluations, which in turn, may enhance functional status.

In addition to our recommendations for monitoring and clinical interventions on an individual and family level, changes also need to be made at a national policy level to facilitate women's adaptation during the childbearing period. The provision of universal paid parental leave during the childbearing year is recommended. Although the Family and Medical Leave Act of 1993 provides for 12 weeks of parental leave following the birth or adoption of a child, a significant percentage of women are excluded from coverage. Specifically, women who work for businesses with fewer than 50 employees or who are in the top 10% of compensated employees of a company are not covered. Also excluded from coverage are women who were not employed for at least 12 months by that employer prior to the leave and women who worked fewer than 1250 hours during the previous 12-month period (Family and Medical Leave Act of 1993, Public Law 103-3).

Although 18 states expanded the benefits provided by federal legislation and have mandated that leave be provided by businesses with fewer than 50 employees (Scheible, 1998), as of 2000 only 58.3% of employees worked in covered establishments (U.S. Department of Labor, 2000). Furthermore, in contrast to the 130 of the 158 countries surveyed that have maternity leave, the United States is one of only four countries— Australia, New Zealand, and Ethiopia are the other three—in which the leave is not paid (Folbre, 2001; Kamerman, 2000). In the United States, only five states and one territory (California, Hawaii, New Jersey, New York, Rhode Island, and Puerto Rico) have paid maternity leave. These states fund maternity leave through their longstanding state temporary disability programs, which expanded coverage to childbearing under the Pregnancy Discrimination Act of 1978. In these states, leaves are funded under the context of pregnancy as a temporary medical disability and, therefore, fathers are not eligible for paid leave (Lenoff et al., 2001). Given that more than half (55%) of all women with a child less than one year of age are in the labor force (Bachu & O'Connell, 2001), universal paid parental leave for childbearing families would enable new mothers to take better care of themselves during the postpartum period and also allow fathers to provide the social support and help needed during this time.

Folbre's (2001) work has highlighted both direct and indirect costs of parenthood. Direct costs of raising children include food, clothing, diapers, health care, housing, and education. Indirect costs include giving up potential income when the woman and/or her partner decide to reduce working hours to spend time at home with the children, as well as potential loss of labor market experience, subsequent promotion to a higher paying position, or eligibility for a new position. Parental leave policies that do not take these costs into account do not serve individuals or society well.

In conclusion, women perhaps most of all need to be helped to have realistic expectations about the childbearing period. Prior to conception, nurses and other health care professionals should seek opportunities to explain to women how modifications in lifestyle may be required during pregnancy and the first few months after childbirth. In addition, nurses and other health care professionals need to view each woman as an individual, encourage her to talk about her particular experiences of adaptation during pregnancy and the postpartum, and listen closely to what she has to say.

REFERENCES

Bachu, A., & O'Connell, M. (2001) Fertility of American women: June 2000. *Current Population Reports,* P20–543RV. Washington, DC: U.S. Census Bureau.

Beck, C. T., & Gable, R. K. (2000). Postpartum Depression Screening Scale: Development and psychometric testing. *Nursing Research, 49,* 272–282.

Beck, C. T., & Gable, R. K. (2001). Further validation of the Postpartum Depression Screening Scale. *Nursing Research, 50,* 155–164.

Family and Medical Leave Act of 1993 (Public Law 103-3). Retrieved January 26, 2002 from http://www.dol.gov/dol/esa/public/regs/statutes/whd/fmla.htm.

Fawcett, J., Tulman, L., & Myers, S. T. (1988). Development of the Inventory of Functional Status after Childbirth. *Journal of Nurse-Midwifery, 33,* 252–260.

Fawcett, J., & York, R. (1986). Spouses' physical and psychological symptoms during pregnancy and the postpartum. *Nursing Research, 35,* 144–148.

Folbre, N. (2001). *The invisible heart: Economics and family values.* New York: The New Press.

Gottesman, M. M. (1992). Maternal adaptation to pregnancy among adult early, middle, and late childbearers: Similarities and differences. *Maternal-Child Nursing Journal, 20,* 93–110.

Kamerman, S. B. (2000). Parental leave policies: An essential ingredient in early childhood education and care policies. *Social Policy Report, 15,* 3–15.

Lederman, R. P. (1984). *Psychosocial adaptation in pregnancy: Assessment of seven dimensions of maternal development.* Englewood Cliffs, NJ: Prentice-Hall.

Lederman, R. P. (1996). *Psychosocial adaptation in pregnancy: Assessment of seven dimensions of maternal development* (2nd ed.). New York: Springer Publishing.

Lederman, R. P., Lederman, E., Work, B. A., Jr., & McCann, D. S. (1979). Relationship of psychological factors in pregnancy to progress in labor. *Nursing Research, 28,* 94–97.

Lederman, R. P., Weingarten, C. G., & Lederman, E. (1981). Postpartum Self-Evaluation Questionnaire: Measure of maternal adaptation. In R. P. Lederman, B. S. Raff, & P. Carroll (Eds.), *Perinatal parental behavior: Nursing research and implications* (Birth Defects: Original Article Series, Vol. 17, No. 6, pp. 201–231). New York: Alan R. Liss.

Lenoff, D. R., Bell, L., Casta, N., Grant, J., Peterman, K., & Rubiner, L. (2001) *Family leave benefits: A menu of policy models for state and local policy leaders.* National Partnership for Women & Families. Retrieved January 13, 2002 from *http://www.nationalpartnership.org*

Mayberry, L. J. (1992). The impact of the marital relationship and infant temperament on symptom distress in the postpartum period. *Dissertation Abstracts International, 53,* 3402B.

McVeigh, C. A., Baafi, M., & Williamson, M. (2002). Functional status after fatherhood: An Australian study. *Journal of Obstetric, Gynecological, and Neonatal Nursing, 31,* 165–171.

Mercer, R. T. (1995). *Becoming a mother: Research on maternal identity from Rubin to the present.* New York: Springer Publishing.

Newton, N. (1955). *Maternal emotions: A study of women's feelings toward menstruation, pregnancy, childbirth, breast feeding, infant care, and other aspects of their femininity.* New York: Paul B. Hoeber.

Roy, C. (1984). *Introduction to nursing: An adaptation model* (2nd ed.). Englewood Cliffs, NJ: Prentice-Hall.

Roy, C., & Andrews, H. A. (1999). *The Roy Adaptation Model* (2nd ed.). Stamford, CT: Appleton and Lange.

Sagrestano, L. M., Rodriguez, A. C., Carroll, D., Bieniarz, A., Greenberg, A., Castro, L., & Nuwayhid, B. (2002). A comparison of standardized measures of psychosocial variables with single-item screening measures used in an urban obstetric clinic. *Journal of Obstetric, Gynecological, and Neonatal Nursing, 31,* 147–155.

Scheible, P. (1998). Unpaid family leave. *Compensation and Working Conditions Online, 3*(4). Retrieved on January 13, 2002 from *http://www.bls.gov/opub/cwc/cwcwelc.htm.*

Tulman, L., Higgins, K., Fawcett, J., Nunno, C., Vansickel, C., Haas, M. B., & Speca, M. M. (1991). The Inventory of Functional Status-Antepartum Period: Development and testing. *Journal of Nurse-Midwifery, 36,* 117–123.

U.S. Department of Labor. (2000). *Balancing the needs of families and employers: The family and medical leave surveys 2000 update.* Retrieved January 26, 2002 from *http://www.dol.gov/asp/fmla/main2000.htm.*

Part V

CONCLUSION

10

Revisiting the Theory of Adaptation During Childbearing

In this final chapter, we summarize the results of our study and discuss how the findings supported our Theory of Adaptation During Childbearing. We also discuss the utility and credibility of the Roy Adaptation Model for research with childbearing women.

CHANGES IN FUNCTIONAL STATUS, PHYSICAL HEALTH, PSYCHOSOCIAL HEALTH, AND FAMILY RELATIONSHIPS DURING PREGNANCY AND THE POSTPARTUM

As explained in chapter 1, the Roy Adaptation Model proposes that changes in stimuli are associated with changes in responses. Accordingly, our Theory of Adaptation During Childbearing proposed that functional status, physical health, psychosocial health, and family relationships all change during pregnancy and the postpartum. The collective quantitative results of our study, as presented in chapters 2 through 7, revealed a somewhat more parsimonious version of the theory.

More specifically, we found evidence of changes in overall functional status across the three trimesters of pregnancy and throughout the first six postpartum months (see Tables 2.1 and 5.1, Figure 10.1 [A1]). We also found evidence of changes in the level of physical energy across the three trimesters of pregnancy and throughout the first six months after delivery (see Tables 2.1 and 5.1, Figure 10.1 [A2]). In contrast, we found no evidence of a change in the number of physical symptoms from the first to the second trimester of pregnancy, although the results indicated changes from the second to the third trimester and throughout the first six months postpartum (see Tables 2.1 and 5.1, Figure 10.1 [A3]).

Furthermore, we found changes only in certain psychosocial health variables, including psychological symptoms, and in certain family relationship variables during the three trimesters of pregnancy and the

Roy Adaptation Model:

Changes in Stimuli   ⟶   Changes in Responses

Theory of Adaptation During Childbearing:

Progression of the Pregnancy   ⟶   Changes in Functional
and the Postpartum   Status, Physical Health
                                               Psychosocial Health
                                               Family Relationships

A1: Functional Status

Study Variables:
First to Second to Third Trimester of   ⟶   Changes in Functional
Pregnancy; 3 Weeks to 6 Weeks to 3   Status
Months to 6 Months Postpartum

A2: Physical Energy

Study Variables:
First to Second to Third Trimester of   ⟶   Changes in Physical
Pregnancy; 3 Weeks to 6 Weeks to 3   Energy
Months to 6 Months Postpartum

A3: Physical Symptoms

Study Variables:
Second to Third Trimester of   ⟶   Changes in Physical
Pregnancy; 3 Weeks to 6 Weeks   Symptoms
to 3 Months to 6 Months Postpartum

B1: Feeling Anxious

Study Variables:
Second to Third Trimester of   ⟶   Changes in Feeling
Pregnancy; 3 Weeks to 6 Weeks   Anxious
to 3 Months Postpartum

B2: Feeling Better Than Usual

Study Variables:
First to Second Trimester of   ⟶   Changes in Feeling
Pregnancy   Better Than Usual

C1: Acceptance of Pregnancy

Study Variables:
First to Second Trimester of   ⟶   Changes in
Pregnancy   Acceptance of Pregnancy

C2: Feeling Prepared for Labor

Study Variables:
Second to Third Trimester of   ⟶   Changes in Preparation
Pregnancy   for Labor

C3: Relationship with Husband

Study Variables:
First to Second Trimester of   ⟶   Changes in Relationship
Pregnancy   with Husband

FIGURE 10.1   **Diagrams of first Roy Adaptation Model proposition, first theory proposition, and study variables: Results after testing.**

D1: Gratification with Labor and Delivery

Study Variables:
3 Weeks to 6 Weeks Postpartum ⟶ Changes in Gratification
with Labor and Delivery

D2: Satisfaction with Motherhood

Study Variables:
6 Weeks to 3 Months Postpartum ⟶ Changes in Satisfaction
with Motherhood

**D3: Maternal Confidence in Ability to
Cope with Tasks of Motherhood**

Study Variables:
3 Weeks to 6 Weeks to ⟶ Changes in Maternal Confidence in
3 Months Postpartum Ability to Cope with Tasks of Motherhood

**D4: Maternal Perception of Father
Participation in Child Care**

Study Variables:
3 Weeks to 6 Weeks Postpartum ⟶ Changes in Maternal Perception
of Father Participation in Child Care

**D5: Maternal Perception of
Infant Temperament—
Fussy-Difficult**

Study Variables:
3 Weeks to 6 Weeks to ⟶ Changes in Maternal Perception of
3 Months Postpartum Infant Temperament—
Fussy-Difficult

**D6: Maternal Perception of Infant
Temperament—Dull**

Study Variables:
3 Weeks to 6 Weeks to ⟶ Changes in Maternal Perception of
3 Months Postpartum Infant Temperament—Dull

**D7: Maternal Perception of Infant
Temperament—Unpredictable**

Study Variables:
3 Weeks to 6 Weeks to ⟶ Changes in Maternal Perception of
3 Months to 6 Months Postpartum Infant Temperament—Unpredictable

**D8: Maternal Perception of Infant
Temperament—Unadaptable**

Study Variables:
3 Months to 6 Months Postpartum ⟶ Changes in Maternal Perception of
Infant Temperament—Unadaptable

D9: Infant Nocturnal Sleep

Study Variables:
3 Weeks to 6 Weeks to ⟶ Changes in Infant Nocturnal Sleep
3 Months Postpartum

FIGURE 10.1   *(continued)*

first six months after delivery. We were left with a considerably more parsimonious version of this part of our theory than we had originally proposed. Specifically, we found evidence of changes in just two of the three psychological symptoms we measured. Anxiety changed only from the second to the third trimester of pregnancy, and from three weeks to six weeks to three months postpartum (see Tables 4.1 and 7.1, Figure 10.1 [B1]). In addition, we found that feeling better than usual changed only from the first to the second trimester of pregnancy (see Table 4.1, Figure 10.1 [B2]). We found no changes in depression at any time during pregnancy and the first six postpartum months.

With regard to the psychosocial health and family relationship variables measured by the *Prenatal Self-Evaluation Questionnaire* (PNSQ), we found that acceptance of pregnancy changed from the first to the second trimester of pregnancy (see Table 4.1, Figure 10.1 [C1]), as did the woman's relationship with her husband (see Table 4.1, Figure 10.1 [C3]). Preparation for labor changed from the second to the third trimester of pregnancy (see Table 4.1, Figure 10.1 [C2]). We found no evidence of changes in any other PNSQ psychosocial health variables (identification of a motherhood role; fear of pain, helplessness, and loss of control during labor; concern for well-being of self and baby) or family relationship variables (relationship with own mother).

With regard to the psychosocial health and family relationship variables measured by the *Postpartum Self-Evaluation Questionnaire* (PSQ), we found that gratification with labor and delivery changed from three weeks to six weeks postpartum (see Table 7.1, Figure 10.1 [D1]), as did maternal perception of father participation in child care (see Table 7.1, Figure 10.1 [D4]). Satisfaction with motherhood changed from six weeks to three months postpartum (see Table 7.1, Figure 10.1 [D2]), and maternal confidence in ability to cope with tasks of motherhood changed from three weeks to six weeks to three months postpartum (see Table 7.1, Figure 10.1 [D3]). We found no evidence of changes in any other PSQ psychosocial health variables (life satisfaction) or family relationships variables (social support from family and friends, quality of the marital relationship after delivery).

Furthermore, maternal perception of two dimensions of infant temperament—fussy-difficult and dull—changed from three weeks to six weeks to three months postpartum (see Table 7.3, Figure 10.1 [D5, D6]). Maternal perception of the unpredictable dimension of infant temperament changed throughout the postpartum (see Table 7.3, Figure 10.1 [D7]). Maternal perception of the unadaptable dimension of infant temperament changed from three months to six months postpartum. Finally, infant nocturnal sleep changed from three weeks to six weeks to three months postpartum (see Table 7.3, Figure 10.1 [D9]).

RELATION OF WEIGHT TO PHYSICAL SYMPTOMS, PHYSICAL ENERGY, AND FUNCTIONAL STATUS DURING PREGNANCY AND THE POSTPARTUM

Based on the Roy Adaptation Model proposition that stimuli are related to responses, our Theory of Adaptation to Childbearing proposed that weight, which we regarded as a focal stimulus, would be related to the adaptation responses of functional status and physical health variables, including physical energy and physical symptoms during pregnancy and the postpartum. The results of our study dealing with weight during pregnancy and the postpartum (see chapters 3 and 6) did not support this assertion.

We found evidence only of an association between weight gained during pregnancy and third trimester functional status. There was no evidence of an association between the woman being underweight, overweight, or of normal weight at the beginning of pregnancy and any of the adaptation responses.

All correlations between postpartum weight variables (absolute postpartum weight, postpartum weight loss, and postpartum weight retention) and the adaptation responses of physical symptoms, physical health, and functional status were of low magnitude (see Table 6.3). The data yielded evidence only of an association between the amount of retained weight from pregnancy and functional status and physical symptoms at three weeks after delivery, and with physical energy at six months after delivery. There was no evidence of an association between any other postpartum weight variables and the adaptation responses.

RELATION OF PHYSICAL HEALTH, PSYCHOSOCIAL HEALTH, AND FAMILY RELATIONSHIPS TO FUNCTIONAL STATUS

The Roy Adaptation Model also proposes that the response modes are interrelated, such that responses in any one mode have an effect on, or act as a stimulus for, one or all of the other modes (see chapter 1).

Accordingly, we proposed that physical health and functional status, psychosocial health and functional status, and family relationships and functional status would be related. We reported the Pearson zero-order correlations for those relations in chapters 2 through 7 (see Tables 2.2, 4.2, 5.2, 7.2, and 7.4). In this chapter, we report the results of multiple regression analyses that allowed us to identify the physical health, psychosocial health, and family relationships variables that best explained variation in functional status. A separate multiple regression analysis was done for each trimester of pregnancy and for three weeks, six weeks, three months, and six months postpartum, using only the physical health, psychosocial health, and family relationships variables that were statistically significantly correlated with functional status (see Tables 2.2, 4.2, 5.2, 7.2, and 7.4).

During the first trimester of pregnancy, the variation in functional status was best explained by physical energy; fear of pain, helplessness, and loss of control during labor; physical symptoms; feeling depressed; and feeling better than usual ($R^2 = .33$, $F = 21.41$, $p < .0005$) (see Figure 10.2 [A1]). During the second trimester of pregnancy, the variation in functional status was best explained by physical energy; physical symptoms; fear of pain, helplessness, and loss of control during labor; and acceptance of pregnancy ($R^2 = .23$, $F = 16.37$, $p < .0005$) (see Figure 10.2 [A2]). During the third trimester of pregnancy, the variation in functional status was best explained by physical energy; feeling anxious; and fear of pain, helplessness, and loss of control during labor ($R^2 = .20$, $F = 18.78$, $p < .0005$) (see Figure 10.2 [A3]).

At three weeks postpartum, the variation in functional status was best explained by physical energy, physical symptoms, and satisfaction with motherhood ($R^2 = .34$, $F = 37.27$, $p < .0005$) (see Figure 10.2 [B1]). At six weeks postpartum, the variation in functional status was best explained by satisfaction with motherhood ($R^2 = .04$, $F = 9.733$, $p < .002$) (see Figure 10.2 [B2]).

At three months postpartum, the variation in functional status was best explained by physical energy and physical symptoms ($R^2 = .22$, $F = 30.53$, $p < .0005$) (see Figure 10.2 [B3]). Finally, at six months postpartum, the variation in functional status was best explained by feeling anxious, physical energy, and maternal confidence in ability to cope with tasks of motherhood ($R^2 = .13$, $F = 11.16$, $p < .0005$) (see Figure 10.2 [B4]).

In summary, throughout the three trimesters of pregnancy, level of physical energy and fear of pain, helplessness, and loss of control during

Roy Adaptation Model:

Response Modes   ⟶   Response Modes
    Physiological Mode   ⟶   Role Function Mode
    Self-Concept Mode   ⟶   Role Function Mode
    Interdependence Mode   ⟶   Role Function Mode

Theory of Adaptation During Childbearing:

Physical Health   ⟶   Functional Status
Psychosocial Health
Family Relationships

A1: Study Variables at First Trimester of Pregnancy

Physical Energy   ⟶   Functional Status
Fear of Pain, Helplessness, and
    Loss of Control During Labor
Feeling Depressed
Feeling Better Than Usual

A2: Study Variables at Second Trimester of Pregnancy

Physical Energy   ⟶   Functional Status
Physical Symptoms
Fear of Pain, Helplessness, and
    Loss of Control During Labor
Acceptance of Pregnancy

A3: Study Variables at Third Trimester of Pregnancy

Physical Energy   ⟶   Functional Status
Feeling Anxious
Fear of Pain, Helplessness, and
    Loss of Control During Labor

B1: Study Variables at 3 Weeks Postpartum

Physical Energy   ⟶   Functional Status
Physical Symptoms
Satisfaction with Motherhood

B2: Study Variables at 6 Weeks Postpartum

Satisfaction with Motherhood ⟶   Functional Status

B3: Study Variables at 3 Months Postpartum

Physical Energy   ⟶   Functional Status
Physical Symptoms

B4: Study Variables at 6 Months Postpartum

Feeling Anxious   ⟶   Functional Status
Physical Energy
Maternal Confidence in Ability to
    Cope with Tasks of Motherhood

FIGURE 10.2 **Diagrams of second Roy Adaptation Model proposition, second theory proposition, and study variables: Results after testing.**

labor provided the consistently best explanation for the level of functional status reported by the women in our study. Following delivery, none of the variables provided a consistently best explanation for variations in functional status. Physical energy was, however, a significant variable at three weeks, three months, and six months postpartum. In addition, physical symptoms was a significant variable at three weeks and three months postpartum, and satisfaction with motherhood was significant at three and six weeks postpartum.

UTILITY AND CREDIBILITY OF
THE ROY ADAPTATION MODEL

The Roy Adaptation Model provided a useful structure for our review of the literature and led to the identification of the study variables. Furthermore, the model guided our thinking about women's experiences during pregnancy and the postpartum and led us to our Theory of Adaptation During Childbearing.

We tested the credibility of the Roy Adaptation Model by examining evidence for the proposition that the response modes are interrelated. Recall from chapter 1 that the physiological mode was represented by the physical health variables of physical energy and physical symptoms. The self-concept mode was represented by the psychosocial health variables of psychological symptoms and PNSQ and PSQ variables, the role function mode was represented by functional status, and the interdependence mode was represented by the family relationships variables of PNSQ and PSQ variables, maternal perception of infant temperament, and infant nocturnal sleep.

One source of evidence was our study findings for the proposed relations of physical health, psychosocial health, and family relationships variables to functional status (see Tables 2.2, 4.2, 5.2, 6.2, 7.2, and 7.4). The correlations ranged in magnitude from an exceptionally small effect size of $r = .003$ to a large effect size of $r = .54$ (Cohen, 1988).

Another source of evidence was the correlation matrices we constructed for all study variables. The magnitude of the statistically significant correlations ($p < .05$) ranged from a small ($r = .10$) to a large effect size ($r = .50$) (Table 10.1). During pregnancy, all modes were interrelated except the role function and interdependence modes. The lowest correlations were between the physiological and self-concept modes at all three trimesters, whereas the highest correlations were

TABLE 10.1 Magnitude of Statistically Significant Correlations Between Study Variables Representing the Roy Adaptation Response Modes During Pregnancy and the Postpartum

Time	Response Modes*	Magnitude of Correlations**
First Trimester	P–SC	.13 to .41
	P–RF	.13 to .44
	P–I	.13
	SC–RF	.13 to .32
	SC–I	.15 to .30
	RF–I	—
Second Trimester	P–SC	.14 to .26
	P–RF	.33 to .37
	P–I	.16
	SC–RF	.25 to .34
	SC–I	.14 to .43
	RF–I	—
Third Trimester	P–SC	.13 to .30
	P–RF	.17 to .34
	P–I	.16
	SC–RF	.22 to .28
	SC–I	.17 to .40
	RF–I	—
3 Weeks Postpartum	P–SC	.14 to .44
	P–RF	.18 to .54
	P–I	.14 to .21
	SC–RF	.21 to .32
	SC–I	.13 to .38
	RF–I	.18
6 Weeks Postpartum	P–SC	.18 to .20
	P–RF	.16 to .49
	P–I	.13 to .17
	SC–RF	.22
	SC–I	.13 to .37
	RF–I	.17
3 Months Postpartum	P–SC	.22 to .32
	P–RF	.30 to .42
	P–I	.13 to .26
	SC–RF	.18
	SC–I	.14 to .35
	RF–I	.17

(continued)

TABLE 10.1 *(continued)*

Time	Response Modes*	Magnitude of Correlations**
6 Months Postpartum	P–SC	.16 to .44
	P–RF	.16 to .21
	P–I	.14 to .17
	SC–RF	.23 to .30
	SC–I	.17 to .40
	RF–I	—

*P: Physiological Mode = Physical Health Variables
SC: Self Concept Mode = Psychosocial Health Variables
RF: Role Function = Functional Status
I: Interdependence Mode = Family Relationships Variables
**Sign of correlation coefficients not specified

between the physiological and role function modes at the first trimester and between the self-concept and interdependence modes at the second and third trimesters. During the postpartum, all modes were interrelated at three and six weeks and three months; at six months, all but the role function and interdependence modes were interrelated. The lowest correlations were between the interdependence mode and the physiological modes, whereas the highest correlations were between the physiological mode and the role function (three and six weeks, three months) and the self-concept (six months) modes.

The correlations in our study are similar in magnitude to the correlations between variables representing the four response modes in Chiou's (2000) meta-analysis of the interrelations between the modes. Collectively, the findings of our study add to the accumulating evidence supporting the credibility of the Roy Adaptation Model. The magnitude of statistically significant correlations between variables representing the four response modes indicated that the modes are interrelated but also independent components of adaptation to environmental stimuli.

REFERENCES

Chiou, C-P. (2000). A meta-analysis of the interrelationships between the modes in Roy's adaptation model. *Nursing Science Quarterly, 13,* 252–258.

Cohen, J. (1988). *Statistical power analysis for the behavioral sciences* (2nd ed.). Hillsdale, NJ: Lawrence Erlbaum.

Appendix

STUDY METHODOLOGY

Design

This longitudinal prospective panel study was designed to explore women's health during pregnancy and the first six months following childbirth. A longitudinal panel design was selected in preference to a cross-sectional/short-term longitudinal design because the number of women required for the mixed design would have been prohibitive from a budgetary viewpoint and would have precluded examination of within-subject changes over an extended period of time.

Data were collected at the end of each trimester of pregnancy—at 12 to 14 weeks, 25 to 27 weeks, and 36 to 37 weeks of gestation; and at four points after delivery—three weeks, six weeks, three months, and six months postpartum. The pregnancy intervals were based on the traditional divisions of the prenatal period noted in the literature. Data for the end of the third trimester were collected at 36 to 37 weeks of gestation rather than at 38 to 40 weeks of gestation to avoid losing third trimester data on women who delivered at term but up to two weeks before their due dates. The postpartum intervals were based on data from our previous research (Tulman & Fawcett, 1988; Tulman, Fawcett, Groblewski, & Silverman, 1990), which indicated these are the times when changes in functional status occur after childbirth.

Sample

Sampling Criteria. The sampling criteria required that the women be married, English speaking, over 18 years of age, have no underlying medical problems (e.g., diabetes, chronic renal or cardiac disease) or preexisting factors in their obstetrical histories (e.g., previous premature delivery, history of incompetent cervix) that would classify them as high risk at the time of recruitment during the first trimester of pregnancy. Even given these sampling criteria, we recognized that some of our sample would develop complications during pregnancy or after delivery. Indeed, 50 women developed serious complications during their pregnancies and an additional two were found to have twin gestations. This group of high-risk women remained in the study.

Sample Size. Subject recruitment continued until 250 women who met the sample criteria were enrolled in the study. The overall attrition rate was 8.4% during the one-year course of the data collection for each woman. The overall attrition rate includes 15 (6%) women who voluntarily withdrew from the study and six (2.4%) women who were dropped from the study for obstetrical reasons. Twelve women voluntarily withdrew during pregnancy, and three others withdrew during the postpartum; these women stated that they no longer wished to participate in the study. The women who were dropped from the study included five women who spontaneously aborted and one woman whose infant died at four months of age from a rare genetic disease.

Complete pregnancy data were available from 227 women. In addition to the 12 women who voluntarily withdrew during pregnancy and the five women who spontaneously aborted, third trimester data could not be collected from five of the six women who delivered prematurely and from one woman for whom a home visit could not be scheduled prior to her term delivery.

Complete postpartum data were available from 226 women. The six women who did not provide third trimester data returned to the study during the postpartum. However, in addition to the 15 women who voluntarily withdrew, the five women who spontaneously aborted, and the one woman whose infant died, three additional women were pregnant again by six months postpartum and, therefore, could not be included in the postpartum data analysis.

Sample Characteristics. The mean age of the women was 30.8 years (SD = 4.2, range = 19–41). All had completed high school, and 68% were college graduates. The women's occupations were: homemaker (13%), sales/clerical (15%), professional/managerial (58%), student (5%), and other (9%). Seventy-eight percent were employed at the time of recruitment; 59% were employed at six months postpartum. Of those employed at the time of recruitment, 61% were employed full-time and 39%, part-time. Sixty-five percent of the women reported annual household incomes of over $40,000 per year. Sixty-seven percent lived in suburban towns. Ninety-three percent of the women were White; 4% were African American; 2%, Asian; and 1%, Hispanic. Eighty-two percent had vaginal deliveries, including 3% who had vaginal births after cesarean deliveries (VBAC). Only three infants weighed less than 2,500 grams at birth, although six women delivered prior to 37 weeks gestation. Thirty-nine percent of the women delivered their first child; 44%, their second; 11%, their third; and 6%, their fourth, fifth, or sixth child.

Instruments

The definition for each study variable is given in Table A.1, along with conceptual model and theory concepts and empirical indicators.

Background Data Sheets (BDS) were used to collect baseline information on selected physiological mode physical health variables, the contextual stimuli of maternal demographic characteristics, and an interdependence mode family relationships variable. Physical health variables included weight; parity; type of delivery; prenatal, intrapartal, postpartal, and neonatal complications; medical restrictions; and infant feeding method. Maternal demographic characteristics included age, education, occupation, and employment status; place of residence; household composition; household income; maternity leave and compensation policies of the employer; and job income lost due to childbearing. The family relationship variable was infant nocturnal sleep. Additional data collected included type of childbirth education and the circumstances surrounding delivery.

All variables measured by the BDSs were self-reported. Self-reported weight is considered an accurate and valid method of obtaining weight information (Stunkard & Albaum, 1981; Troy et al., 1995). Self-reporting of the other variables is typical in the behavioral and social sciences.

BDS Form 1 was used to collect first trimester baseline data. BDS Form 2 was used for second and third trimester follow-up data collection. BDS Form 3 was used to collect data at three weeks postpartum. BDS Form 4 was used for six weeks, three months, and six months postpartum follow-up data collection.

The Background Data Sheets are available from Dr. Lorraine Tulman, University of Pennsylvania School of Nursing, 420 Guardian Drive, Philadelphia, PA 19104-6096.

The *Symptom Checklist* (Fawcett & York, 1986) was used to measure the physiological mode response of the number and type of physical symptoms (a physical health variable) and the self-concept mode response of psychological symptoms (a psychosocial health variable). The *Symptom Checklist* consists of 21 physical symptoms (e.g., nausea, and/or vomiting, indigestion, changes in appetite, food cravings) and three psychological symptoms (feel anxious, feel depressed, feel better than usual) associated with childbearing. The women were requested to indicate whether they experienced each symptom, when it began, and how long it lasted. The *Symptom Checklist* was scored by assigning a value of 1 to each symptom experienced and 0 to each symptom not experienced. For the purposes of this study, a count of the total number of physical symptoms and the total number of psychological symptoms experienced at each data collection point was used. The range of possible scores for physical symptoms was 0 to 21, with higher scores reflecting a greater number of physical symptoms. The range of possible scores for psychological symptoms was 0 to 3, with higher scores reflecting a greater number of psychological symptoms. Content validity of the *Symptom Checklist* was initially established through a review of the literature. Subsequently, five women's health nurse practitioners reviewed the symptom list for completeness. Additional items were added following their suggestions. One-week test-retest reliability in a sample of ten pregnant women was .73 (Fawcett & York, 1986). The *Symptoms Checklist* was administered during each trimester of pregnancy and at three weeks, six weeks, three months, and six months postpartum.

The Symptoms Checklist is available from Dr. Jacqueline Fawcett, PO Box 1156, Waldoboro, ME 04572-1156.

The *Physical Energy Scale* (PES) was used to measure the physiological mode response of physical energy (a physical health variable). The PES is a one-item investigator-developed scale that asks the woman, "Have you maintained your usual prepregnant level of physical energy?" The item was rated on a scale of 1 = "not at all," 2 = "partially," and 3 = "fully." Single-item indicators of global ratings of perceptions of a specific concept have been found to be a psychometrically sound method of measuring a symptom or feeling (Youngblut & Casper, 1993). The PES was administered during each trimester of pregnancy and at three weeks, six weeks, three months, and six months postpartum.

The Physical Energy Scale is available from Dr. Lorraine Tulman, University of Pennsylvania School of Nursing, 420 Guardian Drive, Philadelphia, PA 19104-6096.

The *Prenatal Self-Evaluation Questionnaire* (PNSQ) (Lederman, 1984, 1996; Lederman, Lederman, Work, & McCann, 1979) was used to measure the self-concept mode responses of selected psychosocial health variables and interdependence mode responses of family relationship variables. The psychosocial health variables were acceptance of pregnancy; identification of a motherhood role; preparation for labor; fear of pain, helplessness, and loss of control during labor; and concern for well-being of self and baby. The family relationship variables were the woman's relationship with her own mother and her relationship with her husband during pregnancy. Each of the 79 items on the 7-subscale PNSQ was rated on a 4-point scale of "very much so," "moderately so," "somewhat so," and "not at all." Positive items are recoded for consistent interpretation of scores. The lower the score, the more positive the evaluation of the experience of pregnancy. Cronbach's alpha internal consistency reliability coefficients for the subscales range from .75 to .92. The intercorrelations among the subscales range from .06 to .54., indicating relative independence of the scales. The PNSQ was administered during each trimester of pregnancy.

The Prenatal Self-Evaluation Questionnaire is available from Dr. Regina Lederman, University of Texas Medical Branch, School of Nursing, 301 University Blvd, #J-29, Room 3-504, Galveston, TX 7755-1029.

The *Postpartum Self-Evaluation Questionnaire* (PSQ) (Lederman, Weingarten, & Lederman, 1981) was used to measure the self-concept mode responses of psychosocial health variables and the interdependence mode responses of family relationship variables. The psychosocial health variables were gratification with labor and delivery, life satisfaction, satisfaction with motherhood, and maternal confidence in ability to cope with tasks of motherhood. The family relationship variables were social support from family and friends, quality of the marital relationship after delivery, and maternal perception of father's participation in child care. Each of the 82 items on the 7-subscale PSQ was rated on a 4-point scale of "very much so," "moderately so," "somewhat so," and "not at all." Positive items are recoded for consistency in interpretation of scores. The lower the score, the more positive the evaluation of the postpartum experience. Cronbach's alpha internal consistency reliability coefficients for the subscales range from .73 to .90 at six weeks postpartum. The intercorrelations between subscales range from .17 to .74, indicating relative independence of the subscales. The PSQ was administered at three weeks, six weeks, three months, and six months after delivery.

   The Postpartum Self-Evaluation Questionnaire is available from Dr. Regina Lederman, University of Texas Medical Branch, School of Nursing, 301 University Blvd, #J-29, Room 3-504, Galveston, TX 7755-1029.

   The *Inventory of Functional Status-Antepartum Period* (IFSAP) (Tulman et al., 1991) was used to measure the role function mode response of functional status during pregnancy. The IFSAP was directly derived from the role function response mode of the Roy Adaptation Model. The 45 items on the IFSAP are arranged in six subscales: Household Activities, Personal Care Activities, Child Care Activities, Social and Community Activities, Occupational Activities, and Educational Activities. The women were instructed to indicate the extent to which those activities carried out prior to pregnancy were performed during pregnancy. The Household, Child Care, and Social and Community subscale items were rated on 3-point scales of 1 = "not at all," 2 = "partially," and 3 = "fully." The Personal Care, Occupational, and Educational subscales were rated on 3-point scales of 1 = "decreased," 2 = "remained the same," and 3 = "increased." Items on the latter three scales were recoded to combine the "remained the same" and "increased" responses. Certain items are coded in reverse for consistency in interpretation of scores. A "not applicable" code, which is excluded from score calculations, is used for items not engaged in by a woman. Inasmuch as not all IFSAP items are necessarily performed by all pregnant women, a mean score was calculated for each subscale score and for the total score for each woman. The potential range of scores was 1 to 3; the higher the score, the greater the functional status. Content validity, initial construct validity, internal consistency reliability, and test-retest reliability have been established for the IFSAP (Tulman et al., 1991). Internal consistency reliability was calculated by means of subscale item to subscale total score and subscale to total score. The average correlation, using Fisher's z' transformation (Cohen & Cohen, 1975) for items to subscales, ranged from .57 to .87. Subscale to total IFSAP score correlations ranged from .53 to .90. Test-retest reliability over a 6- to 14-day interval was .90 for the total IFSAC with a range of .27 to .93 for the subscales. The IFSAP was administered during each trimester of pregnancy. In this study the item to subscale correlations ranged from .65 to .81 and the subscale to total IFSAP score correlations ranged from .47 to .88 at the first trimester administration.

The Inventory of Functional Status-Antepartum Period is available from Dr. Lorraine Tulman, University of Pennsylvania School of Nursing, 420 Guardian Drive, Philadelphia, PA 19104-6096.

The *Inventory of Functional Status After Childbirth* (IFSAC) (Fawcett, Tulman, & Myers, 1988) was used to measure the role function mode response of functional status during the postpartum. The IFSAC was directly derived from the role function response mode of the Roy Adaptation Model. The 41-item version of the IFSAC used in this study is made up of seven subscales that tap the seven dimensions of functional status after childbirth: Infant Care Responsibilities, Child Care Responsibilities, Personal Care Activities, Household Activities, Social and Community Activities, Occupational Activities, and Educational Activities. Items on the Personal Care Activities, Occupational Activities, and Educational Activities subscales were rated on a four-point scale of "never," "sometimes," "most of the time," and "all of the time." Items on the other subscales were rated on a 4-point scale of "not at all," "just beginning," "partially," and "fully." The 4-point scales were developed because women in our earlier retrospective study (Tulman & Fawcett, 1988) reported that there were differences in the time between when they first began various activities after childbirth and when they regained their previous level of performance of those activities. Certain items are coded in reverse for consistency in interpretation of scores. A "not applicable" code, which is excluded from score calculations, is used for items not engaged in by a woman. Inasmuch as not all IFSAC items are engaged in by all women, a mean is calculated for each subscale score and the total score. The possible range of mean scores for each subscale and the total IFSAC is 1–4. The higher the score, the greater the functional status. Content validity, initial construct validity, internal consistency reliability, and test-retest reliability have been established for the IFSAC (Fawcett, Tulman, & Myers, 1988). Internal consistency reliability was calculated by means of subscale item to subscale total score and subscale to total score. The average correlation, using Fisher's z' transformation (Cohen & Cohen, 1975) for items to subscales, ranged from .51 for the Personal Care Activities subscale to .78 for the Social and Community Activities. The range of subscale to total scale correlations was .23 (Occupational Activities subscale, $n = 15$) to .89. Test-retest reliability over a 4 to 7 day interval was .86 for the total IFSAC with a range of .48 to .93 for the subscales. The IFSAC was administered at three weeks, six weeks, three months, and six months after delivery. In this study the item to subscale correlations ranged from .61 to .77 and subscale to total IFSAC score correlations ranged from .40 to .93 at the three-week postpartum administration.

The Inventory of Functional Status After Childbirth is available from Dr. Lorraine Tulman, University of Pennsylvania School of Nursing, 420 Guardian Drive, Philadelphia, PA 19104-6096.

The *Infant Characteristics Questionnaire* (ICQ) (Bates, Freeland, & Lounsbury, 1979) was used to measure the interdependence mode response of maternal perception of infant temperament (a family relationship variable) during the postpartum. Sixteen of the ICQ items are used to measure temperament in the young infant (Bates, 1984; Bates, personal communication, September 21, 1987). Items are rated on a 7-point scale, ranging from optimal temperament to difficult temperament. The ICQ items are distributed across four independent subscales: Fussy-Difficult, Unadaptable, Dull, and Unpredictable. Each ICQ subscale is scored separately. The Fussy-Difficult, Unadaptable, and Unpredictable subscales are scored by summing the items, with higher scores indicating more difficult temperament. The Dull subscale is scored by summing two items and subtracting the score for one item. Therefore, the potential exists for negative scores, with higher negative scores indicating less dullness. Concurrent validity of the ICQ is supported by correlations of ICQ scores with other measures of temperament (Bates, Freeland, & Lounsbury, 1979). Construct validity of the ICQ is supported by a study of maternal perception of difficult temperament for preterm and full term infants at three and six months postpartum (Gennaro, Tulman, & Fawcett, 1990). Bates (1979) reported Cronbach's alpha internal consistency reliability coefficients for the four subscales ranging from .39 to .79. Gennaro and colleagues (1990) reported Cronbach's alphas ranging from .23 to .69 at three months postpartum and from .24 to .78 at six months postpartum. The Dull subscale has the lowest reliability in all studies. Therefore, we exercised caution when interpreting data from this particular subscale. Test-retest reliability Pearson coefficients for the four subscales at an average of a 30-day interval range from .70 to .47 (Bates, Freeland, & Lounsbury, 1979). The ICQ was administered at three weeks, six weeks, three months, and six months postpartum.

The Infant Characteristics Questionnaire is available from Dr. John E. Bates, Indiana University Department of Psychology, Bloomington, IN 47405.

An *Open-Ended Questionnaire* was used as a semistructured interview schedule to determine the woman's general perspective about her pregnancy and childbirth experience at six months after delivery. This investigator-developed questionnaire consists of open-ended items dealing with various aspects of pregnancy, childbirth, and postpartum recovery. Krippendorff's (1980) content analysis technique was used to derive and quantify categories of responses from the interview transcripts. Simple tallies were used to record "yes" and "no" responses. The unit of analysis for more complex responses was the phrase or sentence that expressed the woman's reports of their childbearing experiences, as well as factors that helped or hindered them during pregnancy and the postpartum. Frequencies and percentages were calculated for each response category. Interrater reliability between two independent coders was determined in two rounds using a different random sample of transcripts from ten women for each round. Final interrater reliability was established at 82.5%.

The Open-Ended Questionnaire is available from Dr. Lorraine Tulman, University of Pennsylvania School of Nursing, 420 Guardian Drive, Philadelphia, PA 19104-6096.

Instrument Selection. The instruments were selected on the basis of their appropriateness as measures of the study variables, their psychometric properties, and time required to complete the entire questionnaire package, with preference given to fewer and shorter instruments that would take less time to complete. It was thought that such a questionnaire package would increase the women's willingness to fill out the questionnaires repeatedly and, therefore, decrease missing data. It is recognized that the decision criteria resulted in selection of one-item measures of psychological symptoms rather than longer inventories. However, the Fawcett and York (1986) study findings revealed adequate convergence of the one item measure of depression on the *Symptoms Checklist* with the scores on the *Beck Depression Inventory*.

Procedure

The women were recruited by the first author (Tulman) and trained research assistants from obstetrical and nurse-midwifery practices. The study protocol was approved by the University of Pennsylvania Committee on Studies Involving Human Beings. Written informed consent was obtained at the time of recruitment in the obstetrician's or nurse-midwife's office or at the beginning of the first visit in the woman's home. Data were collected by the first author (Tulman) or by our trained research assistants, who were graduate students in nursing, in the women's homes at the end of the first, second, and third trimesters of pregnancy and at three weeks, six weeks, three months, and six months following delivery. On rare occasions (less than ten women), data collection for a particular interview was done either at the woman's workplace at the woman's request, or by mail if a woman had moved from the area. The data collectors were trained in clinical interviewing techniques and eliciting health histories. Each woman was followed, whenever possible, by the same data collector to allow a building of rapport (and thereby decrease attrition) as well as to follow up on topics raised by the women. However, because of research assistants' graduations and family difficulties, 64 (27%) women had visits by a second research assistant, and one (0.4%) woman had visits by three different research assistants.

Each home visit was scheduled in advance by telephone at a mutually convenient time. A *Background Data Sheet*, the *Inventory of Functional Status-Antepartum Period*, the *Symptoms Checklist*, the *Physical Energy Scale*, and the *Prenatal Self-Evaluation Questionnaire* were administered at each prenatal visit. A *Background Data Sheet*, the *Symptoms Checklist*, the *Physical Energy Scale*, the *Inventory of Functional Status After Childbirth*, the *Postpartum Self-Evaluation Questionnaire* and the *Infant Characteristics Questionnaire* were administered at each postpartum visit. In addition, the *Open-Ended Questionnaire* was administered as the last instrument at the six-month postpartum visit. Women's responses to the *Open-Ended Questionnaire* were audiotaped. Each home visit took no more than one hour. The women were compensated for their time by a payment of $10 at the end of each of the first six sessions and a payment of $25 at the end of the last session (total payment = $85).

TABLE A.1 Concepts, Study Variables, Definitions, and Empirical Indicators

CONCEPTUAL MODEL CONCEPTS Middle-Range Theory Concepts *Study Variables*	Definitions	Empirical Indicators
ADAPTIVE SYSTEM Childbearing Women	Women who were in the childbearing cycle.	An initial sample of 250 women who were married, English speaking, over 18 years of age, had no underlying medical problems (e.g., diabetes, chronic renal or cardiac disease) or preexisting factors in their obstetrical histories (e.g., previous premature delivery, history of incompetent cervix) that would classify them as high risk at the time of entry into the study.
FOCAL STIMULUS Pregnancy and the Postpartum	The times during pregnancy and the postpartum when data were collected.	Data were collected at the end of each trimester of pregnancy—at 12 to 14 weeks, 25 to 27 weeks, and 36 to 37 weeks of gestation; and at four points after delivery—3 weeks, 6 weeks, 3 months, and 6 months postpartum.

(continued)

TABLE A.1 *(continued)*

CONCEPTUAL MODEL CONCEPTS Middle-Range Theory Concepts *Study Variables*	Definitions	Empirical Indicators
CONTEXTUAL STIMULI Maternal Demographic Characteristics		
Maternal age	Age of the woman in years.	Item on Background Data Sheet Form 1
Education	The woman's level of education, in years.	Item on Background Data Sheet Form 1
Occupation	The woman's occupation.	Item on Background Data Sheet Form 1
Employment status	The woman's current employment status, categorized as full-time, part-time, not employed, looking for employment.	Items on Background Data Sheet Form 1, Form 2, Form 3, Form 4
Place of residence	The woman's place of residence, categorized as city, suburban, or rural.	Item on Background Data Sheet Form 1
Household composition	The number, ages, and relationship to the woman of all individuals living with her.	Item on Background Data Sheet Form 1, Form 2, Form 3, Form 4
Household income	The total amount of income from all members of the woman's household.	Item on Background Data Sheet Form 1
Maternity leave and compensation policies of employer	The employer's benefit package for paid and/or unpaid maternity leave.	Items on Background Data Sheet Form 3
Job income lost due to childbearing	Amount of income lost from not working due to the pregnancy.	Item on Background Data Sheet Form 1, Form 2

TABLE A.1 *(continued)*

CONCEPTUAL MODEL CONCEPTS Middle-Range Theory Concepts *Study Variables*	Definitions	Empirical Indicators
PHYSIOLOGICAL MODE Physical Health		
Physical symptoms	The woman's self-reported number and type of physical complaints common to childbearing.	21 items on the Symptoms Checklist
Physical energy	The extent to which a woman reported that she maintained her usual prepregnancy level of physical energy.	Physical Energy Scale
Prepregnancy weight	Self-reported weight prior to the current pregnancy, classified as underweight, normal weight, or overweight.	Item on Background Data Sheet Form 1 Classification determined by Body Mass Index, calculated by dividing prepregnant weight in kilograms by height in meters squared (wt[Kg]/ht[m²]): underweight, BMI < 19.8; normal weight, BMI = 19.8–26.0; overweight, BMI > 26.0.

(continued)

TABLE A.1 *(continued)*

CONCEPTUAL MODEL CONCEPTS Middle-Range Theory Concepts *Study Variables*	Definitions	Empirical Indicators
Weight gain during pregnancy	Self-reported amount in pounds, as well as the calculated percentage of weight gained, at the time of data collection during each trimester of pregnancy.	Item on Background Data Sheet Form 1, Form 2 Absolute amount in pounds gained, calculated as the difference in pounds between prepregnancy weight and weight at the time of data collection. Percentage weight gain during pregnancy was calculated as weight gain in pounds divided by prepregnancy weight.
Postpartum weight	Self-reported amount in pounds, at the times of data collection during the postpartum.	Items on Background Data Sheet Form 3, Form 4
Postpartum weight loss	Amount of weight lost from each time of data collection to the next time during the postpartum.	Absolute amount in pounds, calculated as the difference in pounds between prepregnancy weight and postpartum weight at 3 weeks, 6 weeks, 3 months, and 6 months.
Postpartum weight retention	Amount of weight retained during the postpartum over prepregnancy weight.	Absolute amount in pounds, calculated as the difference in pounds between weight at 3 and 6 weeks, 6 weeks and 3 months, and 3 and 6 months postpartum.

TABLE A.1 *(continued)*

CONCEPTUAL MODEL CONCEPTS Middle-Range Theory Concepts *Study Variables*	Definitions	Empirical Indicators
Parity	The woman's self-reported number of live births prior to the current pregnancy.	Item on Background Data Sheet Form 1
Minor prenatal, intrapartal, postpartal, and neonatal complications	Complications experienced by the woman during pregnancy, labor and delivery, and the postpartum, and by the infant, that were not life-threatening.	Item on Background Data Sheet Form 1, Form 2, Form 3, Form 4
Type of delivery	The type of delivery experienced by the woman, classified as vaginal, cesarean, or vaginal birth after Caesarean (VBAC).	Item on Background Data Sheet Form 3
Medical restrictions	Advice the woman reported she received from her physician or nurse-midwife to restrict her activities.	Item on Background Data Sheet Form 1, Form 2, Form 3
Method of infant feeding	The method used to feed the infant, categorized as breast, bottle, breast and bottle, solid foods.	Item on Background Data Sheet Form 3, Form 4
SELF-CONCEPT MODE Psychosocial Health		
Psychological symptoms	The woman's self-reported number and type of psychological symptoms common to childbearing.	3 items on the Symptoms Checklist

(continued)

TABLE A.1 *(continued)*

CONCEPTUAL MODEL CONCEPTS Middle-Range Theory Concepts *Study Variables*	Definitions	Empirical Indicators
Acceptance of pregnancy	The woman's response specifically to the pregnancy.	Prenatal Self-Evaluation Questionnaire, Scale 1
Identification of a motherhood role	The extent to which the woman looked forward to assuming a motherhood role and anticipated her gratification from caring for a baby.	Prenatal Self-Evaluation Questionnaire, Scale 2
Preparation for labor	The extent to which the woman felt informed and prepared to cope with the events of labor.	Prenatal Self-Evaluation Questionnaire, Scale 5
Fear of pain, helplessness, and loss of control during labor	The woman's self-estimated ability to maintain control and cope with the events of labor.	Prenatal Self-Evaluation Questionnaire, Scale 6
Concern for well-being of self and baby	Fears the woman may have about complications arising in labor, resulting in injury to herself or her baby.	Prenatal Self-Evaluation Questionnaire, Scale 7
Gratification with labor and delivery	The woman's sense of gratification and accomplishment versus disappointment from childbirth.	Postpartum Self-Evaluation Questionnaire, Scale 3

TABLE A.1 *(continued)*

CONCEPTUAL MODEL CONCEPTS Middle-Range Theory Concepts *Study Variables*	Definitions	Empirical Indicators
Life satisfaction	The woman's satisfaction with her family's financial status, material assets, and size of the home.	Postpartum Self-Evaluation Questionnaire, Scale 4
Satisfaction with motherhood	The woman's pleasure with nurturant activities and her relative preference for a motherhood role versus other roles.	Postpartum Self-Evaluation Questionnaire, Scale 6
Maternal confidence in ability to cope with tasks of motherhood	The woman's doubts about her ability to parent, to interpret her infant's behavior, and to meet the infant's needs.	Postpartum Self-Evaluation Questionnaire, Scale 5
ROLE FUNCTION MODE Functional Status		
Functional status during pregnancy	The extent to which the pregnant woman reported that she continued her usual personal care, household, social and community, child care, occupational, and educational activities.	Inventory of Functional Status-Antepartum Period
Postpartum functional status	The woman's report of her readiness to assume infant care responsibilities and resume usual personal care, household, social and community, child care, occupational, and educational activities.	Inventory of Functional Status After Childbirth

(continued)

TABLE A.1 *(continued)*

CONCEPTUAL MODEL CONCEPTS Middle-Range Theory Concepts *Study Variables*	Definitions	Empirical Indicators
INTERDEPENDENCE MODE Family Relationships		
Relationship with own mother	The closeness, support, and empathy between the woman and her mother.	Prenatal Self-Evaluation Questionnaire, Scale 3
Relationship with husband during pregnancy	Mutuality, support, and communication patterns in the marital relationship.	Prenatal Self-Evaluation Questionnaire, Scale 4
Social support	The amount of support for the maternal role that the woman received from her parents and from her friends and other family members.	Postpartum Self-Evaluation Questionnaire, Scale 7 (parents) and Scale 8 (friends and other family members)
Quality of the marital relationship after delivery	The woman's evaluation of the quality of the relationship with her husband.	Postpartum Self-Evaluation Questionnaire, Scale 1
Maternal perception of father's participation in child care	The woman's perception of the time and interest the father devoted to child care and the pleasure he derived from child care.	Postpartum Self-Evaluation Questionnaire, Scale 2
Maternal perception of infant temperament	Maternal rating of the infant's temperament, in relation to fussiness and difficultness, dullness, unadaptability, and unpredictability.	Infant Characteristics Questionnaire
Infant nocturnal sleep	The time after birth when the infant starts to sleep through the night.	Item on Background Data Sheet, Form 3, Form 4

REFERENCES

Bates, J. E. (1984). *Information on the Infant Characteristics Questionnaire.* (Available from John E. Bates, Indiana University Department of Psychology, Bloomington, IN 47405).

Bates, J. E., Freeland, C. A., & Lounsbury, M. L. (1979). Measurement of infant difficultness. *Child Development, 50,* 794–803.

Cohen, J., & Cohen, P. (1975). *Applied multiple regression/correlational analysis for the behavioral sciences.* Hillsdale, NJ: Lawrence Erlbaum.

Fawcett, J., Tulman, L., & Myers, S. (1988). Development of the Inventory of Functional Status after Childbirth. *Journal of Nurse-Midwifery, 33,* 252–260.

Fawcett, J., & York, R. (1986). Spouses' physical and psychological symptoms during pregnancy and the postpartum. *Nursing Research, 35,* 144–148.

Gennaro, S., Tulman, L., & Fawcett, J. (1990). Maternal perception of preterm and full term infants' difficult temperament at three and six months of age. *Merrill-Palmer Quarterly, 36,* 201–215.

Krippendorf, K. (1980). *Content analysis: An introduction to its methodology.* Newbury Park, CA: Sage.

Lederman, R. P. (1984). *Psychosocial adaptation in pregnancy: Assessment of seven dimensions of maternal development.* Englewood Cliffs, NJ: Prentice-Hall.

Lederman, R. P. (1996). *Psychosocial adaptation in pregnancy: Assessment of seven dimensions of maternal development* (2nd ed.). New York: Springer Publishing.

Lederman, R. P., Lederman, E., Work, B. A., Jr., & McCann, D. S. (1979). Relationship of psychological factors in pregnancy to progress in labor. *Nursing Research, 28,* 94–97.

Lederman, R. P., Weingarten, C. G., & Lederman, E. (1981). Postpartum Self-Evaluation Questionnaire: Measure of maternal adaptation. In R. P. Lederman, B. S. Raff, & P. Carrol (Eds.), *Perinatal parental behavior: Nursing research and implications* (Birth Defects: Original Article Series, Vol. 17, No. 6, pp. 201–231). New York: Alan R. Liss.

Stunkard, A. J., & Albaum, J. M. (1981). The accuracy of self-reported weights. *American Journal of Clinical Nutrition, 34,* 1593–1599.

Troy, L. M., Hunter, D. J., Manson, J. E., Colditz, G. A., Stampfer, M. J., & Willett, W. C. (1995). The validity of recalled weight among younger women. *International Journal of Obesity, 19,* 570–572.

Tulman, L., & Fawcett, J. (1988). Return of functional ability after childbirth. *Nursing Research, 37,* 77–81.

Tulman, L., Fawcett, J., Groblewski, L., & Silverman, L. (1990). Changes in functional status after childbirth. *Nursing Research, 39,* 70–75.

Tulman, L., Higgins, K., Fawcett, J., Nunno, C., Vansickel, C., Haas, M. B., & Speca, M. M. (1991). The Inventory of Functional Status-Antepartum Period: Development and testing. *Journal of Nurse-Midwifery, 36,* 117–123.

Youngblut, J. M., & Casper, G. R. (1993). Single-item indicators in nursing research. *Research in Nursing and Health, 16,* 459–465.

Index

Ability to cope with tasks of mother-
    hood, confidence in, 114
Adaptation after delivery, 67–134
Adaptation during childbearing, the-
    ory of. *See* Theory of adapta-
    tion during childbearing
African American women, in theory of
    adaptation during childbear-
    ing study, 6
Anticipation of delivery, motherhood,
    43–66
  family relationships
    changes in, 56
    functional status and, 50, 56
    during pregnancy, 49–50
  prenatal self-evaluation question-
    naire, psychosocial health
    variables, 48–49
    changes in, 55
    functional status and, 55–56
  psychological symptoms, 43–48
    changes in, 51
    functional status and, 51–55
  psychosocial health
    functional status and, 49
    during pregnancy, 43–49
  study results, 50–57
Anxiety, postpartum, 102–125
Asian women, in theory of adaptation
    during childbearing study, 6
Australia, lack of parental leave policy,
    145

Background Data Sheets, 8, 171
Bottle feeding
  with breast feeding, postpartum
    weight changes, 93
  postpartum weight changes, 93
Breast feeding
  with bottle feeding, postpartum
    weight changes, 93
  postpartum weight changes, 93
Business, leave provided by, 145

Change
  in functional status
    during postpartum, 77–78
    during pregnancy, 24
  in physical energy,
    during postpartum, 78–80
    during pregnancy, 24
  in physical symptoms,
    during postpartum, 78–81
    during pregnancy, 25
  in psychological symptoms,
    during postpartum, 114, 117–118
    during pregnancy, 51
  in weight
    during postpartum, 94–97
    during pregnancy, 36
Child care
  father's participation in, 114
  functional status, postpartum, 78
  help from family, 120–121
  help from friends, 120–121